An Essential
Medical Miscellany

For Sukie

An Essential
Medical Miscellany

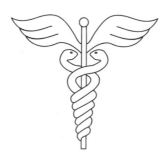

Ayan Panja

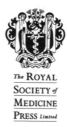

The ROYAL
SOCIETY *of*
MEDICINE
PRESS *Limited*

© 2005 Royal Society of Medicine Press Ltd

Published by the Royal Society of Medicine Press Ltd
1 Wimpole Street, London W1G 0AE, UK
Tel: +44 (0)20 7290 2921
Fax: +44 (0)20 7290 2929
Email: publishing@rsm.ac.uk
Website: www.rsmpress.co.uk

British Library Cataloguing in Publication Data
A catalogue record for this book is available from the British Library

ISBN 1-85315-631-0

Distribution in Europe and Rest of World: Distribution in the USA and Canada:

Marston Book Services Ltd   Royal Society of Medicine Press Ltd
PO Box 269   c/o Jamco Distribution Inc
Abingdon   1401 Lakeway Drive
Oxon OX14 4YN, UK   Lewisville, TX 75057, USA
Tel: +44 (0)1235 465500   Tel: +1 800 538 1287
Fax: +44 (0)1235 465555   Fax: +1 972 353 1303
Email: direct.order@marston.co.uk   Email: jamco@majors.com

Distribution in Australia and New Zealand:

Elsevier Australia
30-52 Smidmore Street
Marrikville NSW 2204, Australia
Tel: +61 2 9517 8999
Fax: +61 2 9517 2249
Email: service@elsevier.com.au

Typeset by Phoenix Photosetting, Chatham, Kent

Printed and bound by Krips b.v., Meppel, The Netherlands

– PREFACE –

'Medicine is universal' – *Sir William Osler*

E very human being has an encounter with medicine during his or her lifetime. The natural processes of birth, death, childhood and ageing are just some of the things that have undergone increasing medicalization as medical science has advanced through the ages. Whether you feel that this is good, bad or ridiculous, it is hard to ignore the importance of medicine's contribution to mankind.

Equally as impressive, if not as important, is the sheer breadth of fact, systems, anecdotes and esoteric minutiae associated with medicine. Some of it is funny. Some of it may be quite disconcerting. Some of it is simply awesome. All of it, however, somehow rouses our curiosity. Why? Because it's about us – the human race, our minds, our bodies and the myriad of things that can happen to us. Whether we like it or not, all of us think about medicine at some point in life, whether it's moaning about a cold or coping with the horror of cancer or a long-term disease.

I hope you will find the book a decent mix of quirky entertainment and information, perhaps an aide-memoire in parts, particularly if you happen to work in healthcare.

For your loo, for your friend the hypochondriac, for your bookcase, for your bedside, for all people and things who are medical, for your information and pleasure – this book is written for them all.

Happy browsing …

– ABOUT THE AUTHOR –

Ayan Panja qualified as a doctor from the Imperial College School of Medicine, London in 1999. He lives in St Albans, Hertfordshire, and is a partner in a medical practice in North London.

– ACKNOWLEDGEMENTS –

Firstly, I would like to give special thanks to Peter Richardson, Alison Campbell and Ian Jones at RSM Press for enabling me to write this unique book. I hope they are all as pleased with it as I am. Thanks also to Mac Clarke for his sterling copy-editing, which has spared me a few blushes.

Individual thanks must also go to Sukie, Shai, Mum and Dad, Bruce, Mr and Mrs JS Gill, Sue Owttrim and Ed Peile, for helping to shape this book in their inimitable ways.

I also owe the following friends thanks for their patience, advice, nudges and suggestions, both sensible and whimsical: Bruce Josyfon, Alice Danczak, Lorna Davitt, Johanna Aspel, Garner Thomson, Niz Eltom, Omar Rahim, Vikram Dhar, Ritesh Sharma, Jon Deere and the many others who have inadvertently put ideas in my head. Thanks finally must go to my friends, old and new, for their support – from Charing Cross & Westminster, Brighton, GP land – and, of course, Bengal.

I would like to take this opportunity to remember and applaud all of the dedicated people who work for the NHS, who continue in their complex daily struggles to help others.

– PUBLISHER'S ACKNOWLEDGEMENTS –

The publisher would like to thank the following for granting permission to reproduce the photographs and text items listed below:

The Royal London Hospital Archives and Museum for the photograph of Joseph Merrick ('the Elephant Man') on page 22; the Isshinkai Foundation, Tokyo, Japan, copyright holders of the Ishihara Tests, for the sample reproduction plates on page 26 – it should be noted that the plates reproduced herein are not appropriate for use in examination of colour sensation; the Wellcome Trust (Historical Collection) for the reproduction of the Florence Nightingale polar area diagram on page 27; the Driver and Vehicle Licensing Agency (DVLA) for the listing on page 56 of medical conditions that must be notified to the DVLA – the list reproduced herein is not exhaustive and is based on the May 2005 guidelines; MedChi, the Maryland State Medical Society, for reproduction of the Barthel Activities of Daily Living Index on page 59; Dr Henry J Heimlich and the Heimlich Institute for details of the Heimlich manoeuvre on page 64; Psychological Assessment Resources Inc, Florida, USA for permission to quote sample questions from the Mini-Mental State Examination by Marshall Folstein, Susan Folstein and Paul McHugh as detailed on page 82; and Dr Meredith Belbin and Belbin® Associates for the list of roles within a team on page 102.

– MEDICINE –

'The art of restoring and preserving health ...'

– A FEW COMMONLY USED MEDICAL ABBREVIATIONS –

	What it stands for	What it means
AAA	Abdominal aortic aneurysm	A bulging of the aorta, which can become weak
ABG	Arterial blood gas	A blood test taken from an artery to check oxygen and carbon dioxide levels
AF	Atrial fibrillation	Irregular, often fast, beating of the upper chambers of the heart
AIDS	Acquired immunodeficiency syndrome	A multisystem syndrome characterized by a weakening immune system
AMA	American Medical Association	A unified voice for American physicians
BMA	British Medical Association	The closest thing to a doctor's union in the UK
BMJ	*British Medical Journal*	A prestigious international medical journal
BNF	*British National Formulary*	The seminal drug guide for British doctors
COPD	Chronic obstructive pulmonary disease	Long-term disease affecting the lungs
CRP	C-reactive protein	A blood protein that rises in level with infection or inflammation
CSF	Cerebrospinal fluid	The fluid surrounding the brain and spinal cord
CT	Computerized tomography	Cross section scan using beams of radiation
CVA	Cerebrovascular accident	A stroke (a fault with the blood supply to the brain)
CXR	Chest X-ray	An image of the chest taken by X-ray radiography
DVT	Deep vein thrombosis	A clot within a deep leg vein
ECG	Electrocardiogram	A tracing of the electrical activity of the heart
ECT	Electroconvulsive therapy	Electric shock treatment for the brain (psychiatry)
EEE	Electroencephalogram	A readout of brain waves useful in sleep studies and epilepsy
ENT	Ear, Nose and Throat	Refers to the specialty by the same name
FBC	Full blood count	A blood test that can reveal anaemia and infection

FRCS	Fellow of the Royal College of Surgeons	A former UK postgraduate examination for surgeons
GI	Gastrointestinal	Relating to any part of the gut (from mouth to anus)
GMC	General Medical Council	No doctor can practise in the UK without being a member of this governing body of doctors
HIV	Human immunodeficiency virus	A virus that can lead to AIDS
IV	Intravenous	Through a vein (drug route)
JAMA	*Journal of the American Medical Association*	A prestigious international medical journal
LA	Local anaesthetic	A drug that causes loss of sensation in one area
LFT	Liver function tests	A blood test to check chemicals produced by the liver
MBBS	*Medicinae Baccalaureus*, Bachelor of Surgery	Basic medical degree in the UK (also BMBS, BMChB)
MD	*Medicinae Doctor* (Latin)	Doctor of Medicine
MI	Myocardial infarction	A heart attack or a coronary thrombosis
MRI	Magnetic resonance imaging	An imaging device using a magnetic field
MRSA	Methicillin-resistant staphylococcus aureus	A bacterium found predominantly in hospitals and which can be harmless or harmful
NAD	No abnormality detected	A normal test or clinical examination result
NSAID	Non-steroidal anti-inflammatory drug	Drugs, such as ibuprofen, that are powerful anti-inflammatories but not steroids
PE	Pulmonary embolus	A clot in a lung vessel, usually following a DVT
PO	Per os	By mouth (drug route)
PPH	Post-partum haemorrhage	Bleeding from the womb after giving birth
PR	Per rectum	Via the rectum
RICE	Rest, ice, compression, elevation	Advice given after sprains and strains
USS	Ultrasound scan	A non-invasive test that uses sound waves to produce pictures of the scanned body part
UTI	Urinary tract infection	An infection of the urine

– SOME LATIN TERMS USED IN PRESCRIBING –

prn	*pro re nata* (when required)
nocte	at night
mane	in the morning
bd	*bis die* (twice daily)
od	*omni die* (daily)
stat	immediately
tds	*ter die sumendus* (three times daily)
qds	*quater die sumendus* (four times daily)
qqh	*quarta quaque hora* (every four hours)
ac	*ante cibum* (before food)
pc	*post cibum* (after food)

– SOME E NUMBERS –

E100	Turmeric	E162	Beetroot red
E102	Tartrazine	E171	Titanium dioxide
E104	Quinolone yellow	E172	Iron oxides
E110	Sunset yellow FCF		and hydroxides
E123	Amaranth	E211	Sodium benzoate
E124	Ponceau 4R	E322	Lecithins
E127	Erythrosine BS	E420	Sorbitol
E132	Indigo carmine	E421	Mannitol
E142	Green S	E422	Glycerol

– THE LARGEST HOSPITAL IN THE WORLD –

The largest hospital in the world is the Chris Hani Baragwanath Hospital in the township of Soweto in South Africa. It has 3200 beds and a staff of 6760 and serves a population of 3.5 million people.

– BONES –

There are 206 bones in the body. The longest bone is the femur (the thigh bone) and the smallest is the stapes, in the ear. As a material, bone is as strong as most common metals.

– THE HEPATITIS ALPHABET –

Hepatitis A is a waterborne infection and is excreted in the stool. It can be contracted from contaminated food and water supplies. It is generally non-fatal and there is a vaccine for those travelling overseas.

Hepatitis B is less common than Hepatitis A, but can be much more severe, resulting in death on occasion. It is transmitted by blood, saliva and semen. There is a vaccine available for health-care workers in the UK, and in the USA this is compulsory for school-age children.

Hepatitis C is transmitted via blood and leads to long-term infection. There is no vaccine. Although contaminated trans-fusions are rare, it is the commonest type of hepatitis transmitted through blood transfusion.

Hepatitis D is common in South America and Africa. It needs the presence of hepatitis B in order to reproduce. The vaccine for the latter works well to prevent hepatitis D.

Hepatitis E is waterborne and can be spread from faeces. There is no vaccine for it as yet.

Hepatitis F no longer exists. It was believed to be French in origin, but is no longer in the hepatitis alphabet.

Hepatitis G is thought to be transmitted via blood. It is the most recently discovered form of hepatitis.

– POISONS AND THEIR SPECIFIC ANTIDOTES –

Poison	Antidote
Cyanide	Dicobalt edentate
Paracetamol	*N*-acetylcysteine
Benzodiazepines	Flumazenil
Beta-blockers	Glucagon
Iron	Desferrioxamine
Organophosphates	Pralidoxime mesylate
Arsenic	Dimercaprol (BAL, 'British anti-Lewisite')

– SARS –

Severe acute respiratory syndrome, or SARS, first appeared as an unusual type of deadly pneumonia in November 2002, in Guangdong Province, China. Over the next six months it spread to numerous countries, including Hong Kong, Taiwan, Canada, Singapore, the Philippines and Germany. The virus was traced back to one man who initially infected eight other guests during his stay at the Metropole Hotel in Hong Kong. Scientists have found that SARS is caused by the coronavirus, which usually causes little more than a runny nose. The theory is that the devastating SARS form of coronavirus (affecting humans) mutated from a form that usually affects only animals. Antibiotics were not shown to be effective against SARS. By July 2003 there were 775 deaths worldwide.

– THE WHITE COAT –

The iconic white coat was originally worn by physicians in the laboratory setting in the 19th century. At the time, advances in medicine meant that people were actually starting to survive their stays in hospital. Hospitals had been associated with almost certain death before this point. The white coat gradually became adopted worldwide, its colour being associated strongly with authority and healing. It is still popular throughout the world today. Many medical schools in the USA hold a formal robing ceremony.

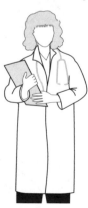

– SOME FAMOUS DIABETICS –

Halle Berry
Paul Eddington
James Cagney
Curtis Mayfield
Mary Tyler Moore
George C Scott
Elizabeth Taylor
Vanessa Williams
Dizzy Gillespie
Ella Fitzgerald
Sir Andrew Lloyd Webber
Elvis Presley
Sir Steve Redgrave
Gary Mabutt
Sugar Ray Robinson
Sir Harry Secombe

– ABDOMINAL INCISIONS AND THEIR NAMES –

Below is a representation of the abdomen and some incision markings.

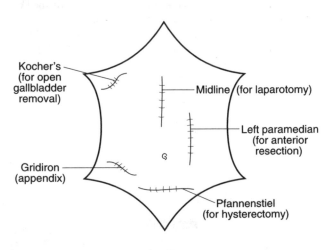

– THE HIPPOCRATIC OATH –

I swear by Apollo the physician and Aesculapius, and Hygiea, and Panacea, and all the gods and goddesses, that, according to my ability and judgment, I will keep this Oath and this stipulation, to reckon him who taught me this Art equally dear to me as my parents; to share my substance with him, and relieve his necessities if required; to look upon his offspring in the same footing as my own brothers, and to teach them this art, if they shall wish to learn it, without fee or stipulation; and that by precept, lecture, and every other mode of instruction, I will impart a knowledge of the Art to my own sons, and those of my teachers, and to disciples bound by a stipulation and oath according to the law of medicine, but to none others. I will follow that system of regimen which, according to my ability and judgment, I consider for the benefit of my patients, and abstain from whatever is deleterious and mischievous. I will give no deadly medicine to any one if asked, nor suggest any such counsel; and in like manner I will not give to a woman a pessary to produce abortion. With purity and with holiness I will pass my life and practise my Art. I will not cut persons labouring under the stone, but will leave this to be done by men who are practitioners of this work. Into whatever houses I enter, I will go into them for the benefit of the sick, and will abstain from every voluntary act of mischief and corruption; and, further, from the seduction of females or males, of freemen and slaves. Whatever, in connection with my professional service, or not in connection with it, I see or hear, in the life of men, which ought not to be spoken of abroad, I will not divulge, as reckoning that all such should be kept secret. While I continue to keep this Oath unviolated, may it be granted to me to enjoy life and the practice of the Art, respected by all men, in all times. But should I trespass and violate this Oath, may the reverse be my lot.

– LISTERINE® –

Listerine® mouthwash is named after the surgeon Joseph Lister (later Lord Lister) for his work on antiseptics. Listerine® is a registered trademark.

– SOME FACTS ABOUT EXERCISE –

Exercise …
… causes the release of endorphins, which improve mood and reduce the chance of depression.
… has recently been shown to be better at preventing diabetes compared with a drug that is used to treat diabetes.
… improves bone density.
… reduces the chance of heart disease.
… improves sleep, concentration and libido.

– THE STETHOSCOPE –

The stethoscope is one of the most identifiable pieces of medical equipment. It was invented in 1816 by Rene Laennec, a French physician. The flat surface is called the diaphragm and the concave part is called the bell. It works by amplifying sound through vibration and conduction. Laennec's original was a long tube designed for use with one ear.

– TEETH –

We have two sets of teeth during our lifetime. There are 20 deciduous ('milk') teeth, which usually develop between the ages of 6 months and 2 years. This set of teeth is lost any time after the age of 6 years and is replaced by 32 permanent teeth: 8 incisors, which cut; 4 canines, which are pointed; 8 premolars, which have cusps; and 12 molars, which grind. Wisdom teeth are the molar teeth furthest back (most posterior).

– ULTRASOUND –

Ultrasound imaging uses sound waves. The sound waves bounce back from the body to an ultrasound scanner. They are then shown as images on a screen. Because ultrasound imaging does not employ potentially harmful radiation, it is safe to use in pregnancy. It is also used for looking at various body parts such as the kidneys, testicles, ovaries and liver.

– NOTIFIABLE DISEASES –

In the UK, a doctor who suspects that a patient may be suffering from one of the following diseases must notify their local consultant for communicable disease control under the Public Health (Control of Disease) Act 1984:

Cholera	Relapsing fever
Food poisoning	Smallpox
Plague	Typhus

The following diseases must be notified under the Public Health (Infectious Diseases) Regulations 1988:

Acute encephalitis	Ophthalmia neonatorum
Acute poliomyelitis	Paratyphoid fever
Anthrax	Rabies
Diphtheria	Rubella
Dysentery	Scarlet fever
Leprosy	Tetanus
Leptospirosis	Tuberculosis
Malaria	Typhoid fever
Measles	Viral haemorrhagic fever
Meningitis	Viral hepatitis
Meningococcal septicaemia	Whooping cough
Mumps	Yellow fever

– TESTICULAR CANCER –

Testicular cancer is now the most common cancer in men aged 25–35 years. About 1 man in 500 will develop the disease before the age of 50. Treatments are generally effective and survival rates are good.

– TYPES OF INTRAVENOUS FLUIDS GIVEN IN HOSPITAL –

0.9% Sodium chloride	Dextrose saline
Potassium chloride	Gelofusin®
5% or 10% Dextrose	

– SOME REFLEXES –

(A reflex is an automatic response to a stimulus)

Plantar – the great toes go down when the sole of the foot is stroked up its outer edge

Knee – the knee jerk is elicited by tapping the patellar tendon just below the knee cap

Blink – is elicited by moving anything, usually tissue, up close to the eye's surface

Grasp – is seen in babies when a finger is placed on their palms

– HOMEOPATHY –

Homeopathy is based on the principle that minimum doses of drugs are most effective i.e. the more dilute a drug, the more powerful it becomes. A homeopathic drug usually produces symptoms of the disease that it is trying to cure based on the premise that like cures like. Each preparation is first ground up (*triturated*), then repeatedly diluted (*potentized*) and finally shaken vigorously (*succussed*).

– THE MOST COMMON PARASITIC DISEASE IN THE WORLD –

Malaria is caused by one of four protozoa: *Plasmodium ovale*, *Plasmodium falciparum*, *Plasmodium vivax* or *Plasmodium malariae*. It is transmitted into the bloodstream by the *Anopheles* mosquito. Malaria prevention and treatment is becoming more difficult because of increasing resistance to drugs. It is common in Africa, the Middle East, the Indian plateau, South East Asia and South America. There are up to 500 million cases a year globally.

– AROMATHERAPY –

Aromatherapy involves facial and body massage using plant-derived essential oils, each with different but specific effects. They may be applied to the skin or inhaled for their desired effect.

– COUNTRIES WITH HIGH RATES OF TUBERCULOSIS –

Afghanistan
Albania
Algeria
Angola
Armenia
Azerbaijan
Bangladesh
Belize
Belorussia
Benin
Bhutan
Bolivia
Bosnia Herzegovina
Botswana
Brazil
Brunei
Bulgaria
Burkina Faso
Burundi
Cambodia
Cameroon
Cape Verde
Central African Republic
Chad
Comoros
Chile
China
Congo
Croatia
Djibouti
Dominican Republic
Ecuador
Egypt
El Salvador
Equatorial Guinea
Eritrea
Estonia
Ethiopia
French Guiana

Gabon
Gambia
Georgia
Ghana
Guinea
Guinea-Bissau
Haiti
Honduras
Hong Kong
India
Indonesia
Ivory Coast
Kazakhstan
Kenya
Korea
Kyrgystan
Laos
Latvia
Lesotho
Liberia
Libya
Lithuania
Macedonia
Madagascar
Malawi
Malaysia
Maldives
Mali
Mauritania
Mauritius
Moldovia
Mongolia
Morocco
Mozambique
Myanmar (Burma)
Namibia
Nepal
Nicaragua
Niger

Nigeria
Pakistan
Papua New Guinea
Paraguay
Peru
Philippines
Poland
Romania
Russian Federation
Rwanda
Saint Helena
Sao Tome and Principe
Senegal
Sierra Leone
Singapore
Slovenia
Solomon Islands
Somalia
South Africa
Sri Lanka
Sudan
Swaziland
Taiwan
Tajikistan
Tanzania
Thailand
Togo
Tunisia
Turkey
Turkmenistan
Uganda
Ukraine
Uzbekistan
Vietnam
Yemen
Yugoslavia
Zaire (Democratic
    Republic of Congo)
Zambia
Zimbabwe

– SYPHILIS –

Syphilis is caused by the bacterium *Treponema pallidum*. There are three stages: primary, secondary and tertiary. There is usually a genital ulcer in the primary stage, with swollen glands. The secondary stage follows after six weeks and includes rashes, muscle aches and fever. The tertiary stage can occur years afterwards and can affect any organ in the body, often the brain, causing mental health and balance problems. It is diagnosed by blood tests and is treated by penicillin. There is much speculation about whether or not King Henry VIII died of syphilis.

– VIAGRA® –

Erectile dysfunction is the persistent inability to achieve or maintain an erection. Causes include diabetes, high blood pressure, heart disease, depression, prostate disease and smoking. One in 10 men suffers with it. Viagra® (sildenafil) is effective in approximately 70% of cases of erectile dysfunction. It works by increasing blood flow to erectile tissue in the penis by preventing the breakdown of a substance called cyclic guanosine monophosphate (cGMP).

– SOME PHOBIAS –

Phobia	Fear of ...	Phobia	Fear of ...
Agoraphobia	Open spaces	Gymnophobia	Nudity
Ailurophobia	Cats	Heliophobia	Sun
Akousticophobia	Sounds	Hypnophobia	Sleep
Altophobia	Heights	Logophobia	Words
Androphobia	Men	Necrophobia	Death
Anthrophobia	Human beings	Pantophobia	Everything
Arachnophobia	Spiders	Phobophobia	Fears
Belonophobia	Needles	Spermatophobia	Sperm
Bibliophobia	Books	Tachophobia	Speed
Coitophobia	Sexual intercourse	Thixophobia	Touch
Cynophobia	Dogs	Tocophobia	Giving birth
Domatophobia	Home	Zoophobia	Animals

– COMPUTERIZED TOMOGRAPHY –

A CT (computerized tomography) scanner works by emitting beams of radiation. A computer uses the information from the beams to work out the density of the tissues examined. Each set of measurements is effectively a cross-section through the body. The computer processes the results and displays them on a monitor. CT scanning is useful in confirming strokes and tumours and in planning treatment with radiotherapy.

– MALE AND FEMALE STERILIZATION –

	Vasectomy	*Female sterilization with tubal clips*
Time taken	15–30 min	25 min–1 hour
Anaesthetic	Local	General
Setting	GP/clinic/hospital	Hospital
Failure rate	About 1 in 1000	About 1 in 200
Effective	After about 12 weeks	Immediately

– CHILD DEVELOPMENT –

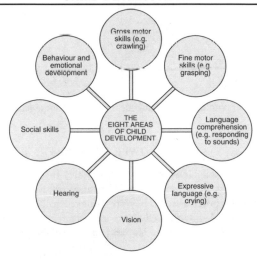

– HEALTH PERCEPTIONS AND MODERN MEDICINE –

A remarkable study by Professor Amartya Sen, Master of Trinity College, Cambridge University, showed that the more a society spends on its healthcare, the more it perceives itself to be sick. The people of deprived Bihar in India have a very low rate of reporting illness, but actually have a high rate of disease and death. It therefore seems incredible that people in the USA are 15 times more likely to report illness than people in Bihar – even though there is far less illness to report.

– PARACETAMOL (ACETAMINOPHEN) –

Paracetamol and its pain-relieving properties were discovered by chance when a similar molecule called acetanilide was given to a patient over a 100 years ago. Its chemical names include *N*-acetyl-*para*-**aminophen**ol and *para*-**acetyl-am**inophenol – hence leading to the derived names acetaminophen in the USA and paracetamol in the UK.

Side-effects include blood disorders and liver damage.

– BACH FLOWER REMEDIES –

Dr Edward Bach (1880–1936) was a Harley Street doctor who devised a system of herbal remedies made from plant extracts mixed with spring water. They are believed to have a positive effect on mood and are used for treating depression and anxiety. They are still in use today and are available from most pharmacies.

– MODIFIED WILSON AND JUNGER CRITERIA –

Wilson and Junger drew up a list of criteria for effective medical screening tests in 1968 – something that the medical establishment still takes note of today. Hence there is, as yet, still no national screening programme for prostate cancer in the UK – mainly because of point 8, here.

1. The condition must be important
2. The natural history of the disease should be well understood
3. There should be a recognizable early stage of the disease
4. Treatment at an early stage should be of more benefit than treatment at a later stage
5. The test must be acceptable to the population
6. The treatment must be available and acceptable
7. The test must be balanced in terms of cost and benefit
8. The test ought to be sensitive (minimal false positives) and specific (minimal false negatives)
9. The process of finding cases ought to be continuous
10. There ought to be a policy on whom to treat

(Wilson JMQ, Junger G (1968) *Principles and Practice of Screening for Disease.* Geneva, World Health Organization)

– AMBULANCE –

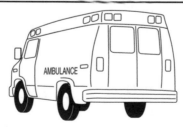

The word 'ambulance' was first recorded in English in 1809. It is taken from the French *hôpital ambulant*: a field hospital or literally 'walking hospital'. This referred to mobile units that followed armies in order to provide urgent medical attention in the field.

– TRIAGE –

'Triage' is a term used in emergency medicine. It is the name given to the process for prioritizing treatment. The word is taken from French, in which *triage* means screening. The noun is from the verb *trier*, meaning to select. Historically, this was applied to the selection and sorting of cattle.

Interestingly, triage in the battlefield was the opposite to triage in modern hospitals – back then, those who were assessed to be the sickest or closest to death were attended to last or left to die.

– X-RAY –

X-rays were discovered by Wilhelm Röntgen in 1895. He noticed that a nearby fluorescent screen started to glow when current was being passed through a vacuum tube. He put this down to mysterious rays, which he called X-rays. X-rays are a form of electromagnetic radiation (like radio waves) and produce an image on photographic film.

– VACCINATION –

It is now more than 200 years since Dr Edward Jenner's first experimental vaccination. This was inoculation with the cowpox virus to build immunity against the deadly smallpox. The word vaccination comes from *vacca*, which means cow in Latin.

– INHALED ANAESTHETICS –

Halothane
Isoflurane
Enflurane } all volatile
Desflurane } liquids
Sevoflurane

Nitrous oxide – 'laughing gas' (commonly used in obstetrics)

– MRI –

MRI (magnetic resonance imaging) is a medical imaging technique that has been used since the early 1980s. There is no exposure to potentially hazardous radiation, as it uses magnetic and radio waves. The patient is placed inside a large, cylindrical magnet that produces a field up to 20,000 times stronger than the earth's magnetic field. Radio waves then cause some of the nuclei of the body's atoms to change their orientation with respect to the magnetic field. When the nuclei return to their original orientation, the MRI scanner detects this, and a computer translates this information into an image. MRI is particularly good at picking up tumours.

– THE RULE OF NINES IN BURNS –

The percentage of the adult body affected by burns is approximated as follows:

1 Palm	1%	Back	18%
1 Arm	9%	Head	9%
1 Leg	18%	Genitals	1%

– TYPES OF SUTURE –

Sutures are the materials used with needles for surgical stitching. Absorbable sutures are used for deep layers, and include:

> Catgut (no longer used)
> Dexon®
> Vicryl®

Non-absorbable sutures are used for minor surgery to close the skin, and include:

> Nylon
> Silk
> Prolene®

The thickness of sutures is reflected by a number – 2/0 being thick and 10/0 being very fine.

– MEDICAL SPECIALTIES AND SCIENCES (A-M) –

Specialty	What the specialty studies, treats or relates to
Anaesthetics	Loss of sensation, pain and consciousness by the use of drugs
Anatomy	Structure of the body
Audiology	Hearing and its assessment
Bacteriology	Bacterial infections
Biochemistry	Chemicals in the body
Cardiology	Heart and heart disease
Cardiothoracics	Surgery to the heart and chest
Community Medicine	Prevention and treatment of disease in the community
Dermatology	Skin diseases
Embryology	Development from conception to about 20 weeks' gestation
Endocrinology	Glands and hormones
ENT	Ear, nose and throat diseases and surgery
Epidemiology	Epidemics and spread of disease
Forensic Medicine	Medical knowledge in detecting crime; crime causing illness
Gastroenterology	Stomach and intestines
General Practice	Family doctor and healthcare team
Genetics	Inherited diseases
Genitourinary Medicine	Sexual health
Geriatrics	The elderly
Gerontology	Ageing and the elderly
Gynaecology	Female reproductive health
Haematology	Blood diseases
Histopathology	Microscopic cell architecture and disease
Immunology	The body and its cells' reaction to foreign stimuli
Microbiology	Bacteria, viruses, communicable diseases

– MEDICAL SPECIALTIES AND SCIENCES (N-Z) –

Specialty	What the specialty studies, treats or relates to
Nephrology	Kidney disease and failure
Neurology	Brain and nervous system
Neurosurgery	Surgery on the brain and nervous system
Nuclear medicine	Radioactive treatments
Obstetrics	Pregnancy and birth
Oncology	Cancer
Ophthalmology	Eye disease and surgery
Orthopaedics	Bone diseases, joint replacements and fractures
Otorhinolaryngology	= ENT (see above)
Paediatrics	Children
Pathology	The causes and natural history of diseases
Pharmacology	Drugs
Physiology	Normal function of the human body
Physiotherapy	Treatment by physical medicine (exercise, etc.)
Plastics	Reconstruction of parts of the body
Proctology	Rectum
Psychiatry	Mental health
Psychology	The mind
Radiology	Imaging of the body using X-rays, MRI, CT scanners, etc.
Radiotherapy	Treatment involving X-rays or other radiation
Rheumatology	Joints and connective tissue
Surgery	Treatment involving operations
Urology	Kidney and urinary tract (surgical)
Virology	Viruses

– SMOKING –

Smoking is the largest single cause of illness and death in the UK. Fortunately, it is completely avoidable and some of its effects on health are totally reversible.

– SOME DRUGS AND THEIR NATURAL ORIGINS –

Drug	Source
Atropine	Belladonna
Colchicine	Autumn crocus
Digoxin (digitalis)	Foxglove
Morphine	Poppy seeds
Aspirin	Bark of willow trees
Taxol® (paclitaxel)	Yew trees
Vincristine	Periwinkle

– CALCULATING BODY MASS INDEX –

$$\frac{\text{Weight (kg)}}{\text{Height (m}^2)} = \text{Body Mass Index (BMI)}$$

BMI < 18.5	is considered underweight
BMI 18.5 – 24.9	is considered healthy
BMI 25 – 29.9	is considered overweight
BMI 30 – 39.9	is considered obese
BMI > 40	is considered morbidly obese

– SIR ARTHUR CONAN DOYLE –

Sir Arthur Conan Doyle was born on 22 May 1859 in Edinburgh, Scotland. After gaining a medical degree at the University of Edinburgh, he joined a medical practice in Southsea, Hampshire, where he also began writing. He soon created the character of Sherlock Holmes, the world-famous detective. Holmes was modelled on a charismatic physician named Dr Joseph Bell whom Conan Doyle had met while at medical school. Conan Doyle was knighted before his death in 1930.

– PENICILLIN –

One of the most important antibiotics in the world was discovered by accident by Sir Alexander Fleming in 1928. He was working on the influenza virus, and noticed that mould had developed on a culture plate for bacteria called staphylococci and that there was a bacteria-free circle around it. He cultured the mould and found that it prevented the bacteria from growing. He christened this active ingredient penicillin.

– CHOLESTEROL –

Cholesterol is a fatty substance that is made mainly by the liver. Not all cholesterol is bad for us. There are two types, which together make up 'total cholesterol'. They are *HDL* (high-density lipoprotein) cholesterol and *LDL* (low-density lipoprotein) cholesterol. HDL protects the heart and LDL increases the risk of heart disease. Thus, a fit athlete may have a very high total cholesterol level because of high levels of HDL.

– INFLUENZA –

Influenza or 'flu is a virus that usually causes fever, muscle ache, sore throat and cough. In 1918 there were 21 million deaths from the influenza virus. Influenza can change with time and there are many types. Hence vaccination does not necessarily give protection in the long term.

– JOHN BODKIN ADAMS –

Dr John Bodkin Adams was a GP who lived in the Sussex town of Eastbourne. He was a beneficiary in 132 of his patients' wills, through which he gathered expensive cars, antique jewellery and almost £50,000. He was acquitted of the murder of a wealthy lady called Edith Morrell in 1957 and remarkably went on to practise until retirement. He also spent a short spell as a teacher at Brighton College, a public school on the south coast.

– GREEN TEA –

Green Tea is made from *Camellia Sinesis*, which contains a chemical called catechin. This has been shown to:

> … reduce the risk of prostate cancer
> … reduce the overall risk of heart disease
> … reduce cholesterol levels

– THE ELEPHANT MAN –

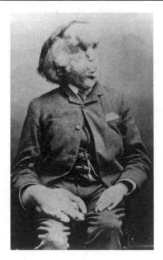

Joseph Merrick (the Elephant Man), was born on 5 August 1862 in Leicester, England. His development as a child was not unusual until about the age of two, when small growths began to appear on his head. These were operated on in his teenage years. It wasn't until he was in his twenties that he was first presented as 'the Elephant Man' at various 'freak shows'. A physician called Dr Frederick Treves looked after him until his death at the age of 27. There is much speculation as to his actual medical condition, which is now thought to be a very rare condition called Proteus syndrome, which involves the overgrowth of tissues. Joseph Merrick wrote much prose and poetry about his life.

– ALEXANDER TECHNIQUE –

The Alexander Technique is a process of retraining in posture, balance and breathing. This leads to a sense of physical and mental well-being, inner tranquillity and confidence. It was developed by F Matthias Alexander, who wrote *The Use of Self* in 1932.

– FAMOUS FIGURES IN MYTHOLOGY, HISTORY AND THE PRESENT-DAY WITH VISUAL IMPAIRMENT OR BLINDNESS –

Helen Keller	Henry Fawcett	Oedipus
David Blunkett	Homer	Samson
Louis Braille	John Milton	St Paul
Ray Charles	Claude Monet	Tiresias
Cupid/Eros	Horatio Nelson	Stevie Wonder
Eduard Degas		

– HARLEY STREET –

Harley Street in central London is famous for its reputation for being the home of England's (and some of the world's) leading private doctors. Indeed, many leading specialists have consulting rooms with this address. Unfortunately, the Harley Street name is not a guarantee of excellence. It is possible for consulting rooms to be rented by almost anyone wishing to do so.

– ACUPUNCTURE –

Acupuncture is an ancient Chinese system of medicine based on the belief that health is dependent on internal harmony. It is expressed through *Yin*, *Yang* and *Chi*. *Yin* is a passive force and *Yang* is a positive force. *Chi* is the 'life force' and is concentrated along 12 pairs of meridians (or channels), along with two single meridians. If these points are stimulated, either by fine needles or a dried herb called moxibustion, the flow of *Chi* can be improved, thereby relieving illness. Acupuncture is widely used in the relief of pain, particularly in the Far East, but also increasingly in the West. It can be used for a variety of conditions apart from pain relief.

– VITAMINS –

Vitamin	Benefits	Sources
A (retinol)	Prevents childhood infections and night blindness	Carrots, liver
B1 (thiamin)*	Prevents damage to the brain, the heart and the nerves	Wheat, nuts
B2 (riboflavin)*	Prevents skin problems	Milk, broccoli
B6 (pyridoxine)*	Keeps blood vessels and nervous tissue healthy	Bananas, cereals
B12 (cobalamin)*	Keeps the nervous system healthy	Eggs, poultry
Niacin*	Made in the body as well as absorbed from foods	Eggs, cheese
Pantothenic acid*	Maintains healthy brain function	Poultry, eggnog
Biotin*	Helps metabolism	Numerous
Folate*	Prevents neural tube defects at birth	Beetroot, peas
C (ascorbic acid)	Keeps connective tissue and immune system healthy	Citrus fruits
D (cholecalciferol)	Keeps bones nourished	Oily fish, eggs
E (tocopherol)	Keeps skin and reproductive organs healthy	Cereals, nuts
K	Prevents blood disorders	Leafy vegetables

* These constitute the 'vitamin B complex'

– THE HUMAN INTESTINE –

The human intestine can measure up to 8 metres in length.

– FREUD –

Dr Sigmund Freud was born in Austria in 1865 and was a physician who established the study of the unconscious mind. He studied medicine in Vienna and developed an interest in neurology. Through an interest in literature, he developed methods of interpreting dreams and founded psychoanalytic theory. He described concepts known as id, ego and super ego, which can be used to explain how our minds work consciously and subconsciously. He eventually fled to London in 1939 after the Nazis occupied Austria. He died a year later at his home in Hampstead.

– THE ODDS OF PREVENTING DEATH FROM VASCULAR DISEASE –

A study in 1999 compared the effect of factors that prevent death from vascular disease – a term encompassing heart attacks, strokes and thromboembolism. It showed the following:

The odds of preventing death from vascular disease over the course of 5 years ...

By eating a Mediterranean diet . . are 1 in 9   *Most effective*
By eating oily fish . . . . are 1 in 19
By stopping smoking . . . . are 1 in 21
By taking a statin . . . . are 1 in 26
(cholesterol-lowering drug)
By taking a beta-blocker . . . . are 1 in 30
By taking aspirin . . . . are 1 in 37   *Least effective*

– FIRST HEART TRANSPLANT –

The first ever heart transplant was performed by Professor Christiaan Barnard on 3 December 1967 in Cape Town, South Africa on 55-year-old Louis Washkansky. The operation lasted five hours and the patient survived for 18 days.

– ISHIHARA TESTS –

Colour blindness is an inherited condition. It is 20 times more common in men than in women, and between 10–25% of the male population is colour blind. The table below shows what a person with normal colour vision should see in the pairs of pictures (Ishihara tests), compared with what is seen by someone who is red–green deficient. Colour blindness can affect employment (pilots, train drivers, etc.).

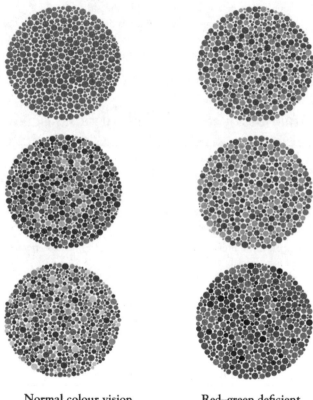

	Normal colour vision		Red–green deficient	
Top pair	12	29	12	70
Middle pair	3	45	5	Spots
Bottom pair	5	Spots	Spots	2

– FLORENCE NIGHTINGALE AND HER POLAR AREA DIAGRAM –

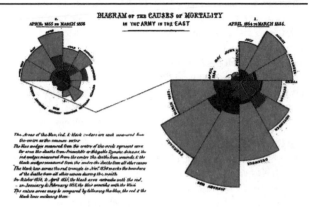

Above is an example of a 'polar area diagram', which was invented by Florence Nightingale and was a way of looking at the causes of army deaths. These were mostly because of a lack of sanitation. The text in the bottom left hand corner of the diagram reads:

'The Areas of the blue, red, & black wedges are each measured from the centre as the common vertex.

The blue wedges measured from the centre of the circle represent area for area the deaths from Preventable or Mitigable Zymotic diseases, the red wedges measured from the centre the deaths from wounds, & the black wedges measured from the centre the deaths from all other causes.

The black line across the red triangle in Nov. 1854 marks the boundary of the deaths from all other causes during the month.

In October 1854, & April 1855, the black area coincides with the red, in January & February 1855, the blue coincides with the black.

The entire areas may be compared by following the blue, the red, & the black lines enclosing them.'

Florence Nightingale's groundbreaking achievements in nursing and in the sanitary reform of hospitals were astonishing, considering that most women in her day did not pursue professional careers. Her father strongly believed that women should get an education and in due course she became particularly proficient at mathematics. She became a Fellow of the Royal Statistical Society in 1858. Many are unaware of her excellence in this field as well as her invaluable contribution to medicine.

– THE ROYAL COLLEGES –

The Royal College of Physicians (RCP) was created by Royal charter of King Henry VIII in 1518. It is the oldest medical institution in England. Its original function was to grant licences to those qualified to practise medicine and to police those engaging in malpractice. It is famous for publishing the *Nomenclature of Diseases* in 1869, which set the standard worldwide for the classification of diseases. This was eventually superseded by the World Health Organization's *Manual of the International Classification of Diseases*. Historically, most of the first British physicians had Oxbridge degrees.

The Royal College of Surgeons (RCS) was created only a few years later, and, since then, with increasing specialization in medicine, there has been the creation of many more Royal Colleges. Many were originally faculties of either the RCP or the RCS. The other Colleges are the Royal College of General Practitioners (RCGP), the Royal College of Psychiatrists (RCPsych), the Royal College of Anaesthetists (RCA), the Royal College of Paedatrics and Child Health (RCPCH), the Royal College of Ophthalmologists (RCOphth), the Royal College of Obstetricians and Gynaecologists (RCOG), the Royal College of Pathologists (RCPath) and the Royal College of Radiologists (RCR).

Membership and Fellowship of the Royal Colleges is generally by examination. They all aim to encourage and uphold the highest standards of medical practice.

– AYURVEDA –

Ayurveda is a system of metaphysical medicine from ancient India. It dates back to 3000 BC and most Chinese and Western medicine is derived from it. Ayurvedic doctors see the body, mind and universe as balanced energies that are in a state of continuous flux with one other. There are seven tissues in the body (*Dhatus*) that, if balanced, ought to create good health. There is emphasis on treating persons as individuals and the use of yogic breathing techniques and healthy diets. Astrology plays a part in diagnosis, and treatment may involve any of the thousands of Ayurvedic drug formulations, which are all natural in origin.

– MENTAL STATE EXAMINATION –

The Mental State Examination is used most often by psychiatrists to assess patients. It consists of the following:

Appearance
Behaviour
Speech
Mood
Thought abnormalities
Hallucinations
Cognition
Insight

– COMPARE SOME 'USUAL' SYMPTOMS OF PREGNANCY … –

Backache

Fatigue

Headache

Insomnia

Nausea

Changeable mood

– … WITH COMMON SYMPTOMS OF DEPRESSION OR ANXIETY –

Backache

Fatigue

Headache

Insomnia

Nausea

Changeable mood

– THE OLDEST MEDICAL SCHOOL IN THE WORLD –

The oldest medical school in the world is Naples Medical School at St Aniello a Caponapoli in Italy. Its origins date back to the 6th century AD. It continues to train doctors today.

– THE GLASGOW COMA SCALE –

This scale assesses a patient's level of consciousness – usually in an emergency setting – by scoring three types of response, which add up to give a total score.

Response		Score
Eye response	Opens spontaneously	4
(one or both)	Opens to verbal commands	3
	Opens to pain	2
	No response	1
Verbal response	Talking and orientated	5
(speech)	Confused and disorientated	4
	Inappropriate words	3
	Incomprehensible sounds	2
	No response	1
Motor response	Obeys commands	6
(movement)	Localizes pain	5
	Withdraws from pain	4
	Abnormal flexion	3
	Extension	2
	No response	1
	Total	**3–15**

(Teasdale G, Jennett B, Assessment of coma and impaired consciousness: a practical scale. *Lancet*, July, 1974, vol ii, 81)

– CANCERS THAT CAN SPREAD TO BONE –

Breast	Renal
Bronchus	Prostate
Thyroid	

– ANATOMICAL PLANES AND TERMS –

All lines and planes are imaginary and are used to describe position.

	Meaning	Example
Median plane	A vertical plane running down the middle of the body	
Sagittal plane	Any plane parallel to the median plane	
Coronal plane	Any plane at right angles to a sagittal plane	
Horizontal plane	A plane running at right angles to the median plane	
Superior (cranial)	Nearer to the head	The eyes are *superior* to the mouth
Inferior (caudal)	Nearer to the feet	The feet are *inferior* to the knees
Anterior (ventral)	Nearer to the front	The nose is *anterior* to the ears
Posterior (dorsal)	Nearer to the back	The ears are *posterior* to the nose
Medial	Nearer to the medial plane	The nose is *medial* to the eye
Lateral	Away from the medial plane	The shoulder is *lateral* to the heart
Proximal	Nearer to the trunk or origin	The elbow is *proximal* to the hand
Distal	Away from the trunk or origin	The toes are *distal* to the ankle
Superficial	Nearer to the surface	Skin is *superficial* to bone
Deep	Away from surface	Muscle is *deep* to skin

– MEDICAL MEANINGS OF WORDS AND HOW THEY ARE PERCEIVED –

	Actual medical meaning	**Common perception**
Vertigo	A feeling of dizziness	A fear of heights
Pneumonia	A type of chest infection, sometimes severe	Always serious, associated with cold environments and death
Chronic	Long-standing or long-term	Serious or severe
Superficial	Not deep to the skin	Not serious
Tumour	Swelling	Cancer
Schizophrenia	A condition affecting thought, often with hallucinations and delusions	Split-personality

– 'CAGE' QUESTIONNAIRE –

This short questionnaire is often used to assess whether someone is dependent on alcohol.

Have you felt you ought to **C**ut down on your drinking?
Have you felt **A**nnoyed by people criticizing your drinking?
Have you ever felt **G**uilty about your drinking?
Have you ever had an **E**ye-opener in the morning?

– RISK FACTORS FOR SUICIDE –

Being male
The risk increases with age
Social isolation
Divorce or separation
Occupation (particularly doctors and farmers)
Depression
Alcohol or drug abuse
Schizophrenia
Serious medical illness

– THE SUN SAFETY CODE –

- Take care not to burn
- Cover up with loose clothing, a hat and sunglasses
- Find shade during the hottest time of the day
- Apply a high-factor sunscreen on parts of the body exposed to the sun
- Be extra cautious to protect children in the sun

– THE STAFF AND THE SNAKE(S) –

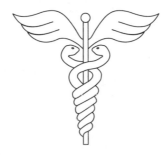

What exactly is the story behind the staff and the snakes and why is there sometimes only one snake? Why are these symbols associated with medicine? Aesculapius was the Roman god of healing, and myth has it that he regarded serpents as special as they were able to renew their youth by shedding their skin. Traditionally, the symbol of Aesculapius bears only one serpent or snake. This is the emblem used by the World Health Organization.

The symbol above (and on the front cover of this book) is called the Caduceus symbol and is a representation of the magic wand of the Greek god Hermes (the same as the Roman god Mercury). The link between this symbol and medicine seems to have arisen from the association of Hermes with alchemy. American health organizations seem to prefer the use of this emblem over the symbol of Aesculapius.

– ENTITLEMENT TO FREE PRESCRIPTIONS IN THE UK –

Prescriptions for contraception

Patients under 16 years and over 60 years or 16–18 years and in full-time education

Pregnant women and women who have had a baby less than 12 months ago

Persons receiving income support, job-seeker's allowance, the guarantee credit of Pension Credit, working families tax credit or disabled person's tax credit

Patients with: Diabetes mellitus that is not controlled by diet alone
Myxoedema
Epilepsy requiring continuous treatment
Permanent fistula needing dressings, etc.
Hypoadrenalism needing replacement therapy
Hypopituitarism and diabetes insipidus
Hypoparathyroidism
Myasthenia gravis
Continuing physical disability preventing going out without help

War and MoD pensioners if the prescription is related to a pensionable condition

Low income and application for any of the above

– HAROLD SHIPMAN –

Dr Harold Shipman was the world's biggest serial killer. As a GP in Hyde in Greater Manchester, over a period of many years, he killed at least 215 of his patients – mostly female. The motive for his killings is still not clear, but he had seen his own mother suffer much pain before her death from cancer when he was 17 years old. He was jailed for life, but hanged himself in Wakefield Prison on 13 January 2004, on the eve of his 58th birthday. His obituary in the *British Medical Journal* was entitled 'Harold Shipman – GP and murderer'.

– BOTOX® –

Botox® is a trade name for botulinum toxin A, which is a toxin associated with botulism. Botulism is a type of food poisoning caused by the bacterium *Clostridium botulinum*, which produces botulinum toxin A. This toxin paralyses muscles and so injections of Botox® are a way of using this paralysing power in areas that may look better – such as frown lines on the face. It is becoming increasingly popular worldwide. The long-term effects of Botox® are still unknown.

– THE FOUR STAGES OF BURNOUT (MASLACH) –

Overwork
Frustration
Resentment
Depression

(Maslach C, Jackson S, Leiter M (1996) *Maslach Burnout Inventory Manual*, 3rd edn. California, Consulting Psychologist Press)

– APGAR SCORE –

The Apgar Score reflects the condition of the newborn baby, by looking at five clinical features. The maximum score is 10.

Features	Scores 0	Scores 1	Scores 2
Heart rate	None	<100 beats a minute	>100 beats a minute
Breathing	None	Weak cry, irregular breathing	Strong cry, regular breathing
Muscle tone	Limp	Some muscle tone	Active movement
Response to stimuli	None	Some expression	Cry, sneeze, cough, etc.
Colour	Pale/blue	Blue at extremeties only	Pink

– FINGERPRINTS –

Fingerprints are impressions left on surfaces made by the ridges on the skin of our fingertips. There are four patterns of ridges: loops, arches, whorls and compounds (a combination of the others). No two people ever have the same fingerprints – and that includes identical twins.

– CANNABIS –

The leaves of the Indian hemp plant *Cannabis Sativa* can be dried and smoked, eaten or drunk. The active ingredient is called THC (tetrahydrocannabinol). It creates a subjective feeling of relaxation. It also causes a dry mouth and an increased appetite. Large doses can cause paranoia and psychosis. Prolonged regular use can lead to apathy.

– NORMAL BODY TEMPERATURE –

The normal body temperature should be around 37 °C.

– ACHILLES TENDON –

The function of the Achilles tendon is to raise the heel. Sudden stretching can cause it to rupture. Its name comes from Greek mythology. When Achilles was born, his mother dipped him into the magical river Styx with the hope of making him immortal. She did this by holding him by his heel, which remained untouched by the river's special water, thus remaining vulnerable – hence the term Achilles heel.

– SOME SCREEN AND STAGE SHOWS NAMED AFTER FICTIONAL DOCTORS –

Doctor Zhivago (1965)   Dr Kildare (1961)
Dr Dolittle (1967)   Doktor Faustus (1982)
Dr No (1962)   Dr Jack (1922)
Doctor Who (1963)

– SOME FAMOUS DOCTORS FROM THE BIG AND SMALL SCREEN –

Dr Michaela Quinn . . . . Jane Seymour
(*Dr Quinn, Medicine Woman*)
Dr Doug Ross (*ER*) . . . . George Clooney
Dr R Quincy (*Quincy*) . . . . Jack Klugman
Sir Lancelot Spratt . . . . James Robertson Justice
(*Doctor in Distress*)
Dr Finlay (*Dr Finlay's Casebook*) . . . . . Bill Simpson
Dr Tom Latimer (*Don't Wait Up*) . . . . Nigel Havers
Dr Mark Sloan (*Diagnosis Murder*) . . . Dick Van Dyck
Captain Benjamin Franklin . . . . Alan Alda
'Hawkeye' Pierce (*M*A*S*H*)
Dr Tony Garcia (*Young Doctors*) . . . . . Tony Alvarez
Mr Anton Mayer (*Holby City*) . . . . . . George Irving
Dr Gregory House (*House*) . . . . Hugh Laurie

– EPILEPSY – A CONDITION OF GREATNESS? –

The following historical figures had, or are thought to have had, epilepsy:

Julius Caesar   Leonardo da Vinci
Alexander the Great   Sir Isaac Newton
Vincent Van Gogh   Charles Dickens
Peter the Great   Peter Tchaikovsky
Vladimir Lenin   Sir Walter Scott
Pope Pius IX   Hannibal
Napoleon Bonaparte   Michelangelo
Joan of Arc

– PHOSPHENES –

Phosphenes are flashes of light that are seen when a person experiences a blow to the eye or when the eyelid is pressed against the ball of the eye. This occurs as a result of stimulation of photoreceptors. There are certain conditions that can cause the phenomenon, including papilloedema, glaucoma and multiple sclerosis. An interesting cause of phosphenes is when the eye has no optical input such as when a person is in a totally dark room or wears light-excluding blindfold. Once the eye has become accustomed to the darkness, the person can often visually experience light in various colours. This may be the explanation behind prisoners reporting ghosts in dark dungeons and for religious meditations in the dark resulting in 'seeing the light'. Any lack of optical input, not just darkness, can cause phosphenes to occur. Airline pilots, for example, often experience them as they fly through a sky without clouds. Children are thought to be able to create phosphenes more easily than adults.

– AVPU –

AVPU is a quick approximation of a person's level of consciousness

A	Alert
V	Responds to Vocal stimuli
P	Responds to Painful stimuli
U	Unresponsive to any stimuli

– WHISKY MATTERS –

The health-giving properties of whisky have been commented upon since its creation. This is because it contains antioxidants. A study in the *British Medical Journal* found that whisky in small doses can help to protect against heart disease, strokes and cataracts. Moderate drinkers of any kind of alcohol are 30% more likely than teetotallers to survive a heart attack. They also have better health in general, including increased levels of alertness and fewer colds.

– FLAT FEET (PES PLANUS) –

The term 'flat feet' usually applies to both feet, where the arches are absent and the soles rest flat on the ground. Normally, the arches do not form until the age of six, but in flat-footed people, they do not develop at all because of weak muscles or ligaments. Flat feet can also be caused by large weight gain. Rarely, they can be caused by a medical condition, such as poliomyelitis. Usually, no treatment is required for flat feet. If there is pain from walking, arch supports and physiotherapy can help.

– ERNESTO 'CHÉ' GUEVARA –

Dr Ernesto 'Ché' Guevara (1928–1967) was most famed for his role in the Cuban revolution and his commitment to equality for all. As a young child he was largely schooled at home by his mother. This was because of severe asthma attacks that required injections of adrenaline. Indeed it was his asthma that sparked his interest in medicine, and he went on to become a doctor after taking his medical degree at Buenos Aires University.

– COMMONEST CAUSE OF SUDDEN DEATH –

The commonest cause of sudden death, worldwide, is cardiac arrest.

– THE INGREDIENTS OF SAVLON® –

The active ingredients of Savlon® are: cetrimide 0.5% w/w and chlorhexidine gluconate 0.1% w/w. It also contains cetostearyl alcohol, liquid paraffin, methylhydroxybenzoate, propylhydroxybenzoate, perfume and purified water.

– THE IRIS –

The iris is the most active muscle in the body. It moves about 100,000 times a day.

– DNA –

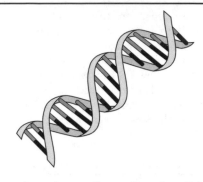

DNA (deoxyribonucleic acid) was first identified in 1869 by Friedrich Miescher. Its structure was proposed much later, by Francis Crick and James Watson in 1953. DNA is a double-stranded molecule responsible for passing on genetic information, and holds information about all of the characteristics of an individual. Everyone has different DNA, with the exception of identical twins.

Advanced scientific technology has made DNA a useful tool in solving crimes (DNA profiling), gene therapy and drug development. DNA technology has even made it possible to analyse blood from the clothes of Abraham Lincoln.

– SOME MAMMOTH MEDICAL MYTHS –

It's bad to reach above your head during pregnancy …

Drinking coffee 'stunts your growth' …

If you cross your eyes too much, they will stay that way …

Going outside with wet hair results in catching a cold …

Tickling an infant's feet will make him/her stammer when older …

Hiccups help you grow …

Cotton buds are good for clearing wax out of ears …

– DNA –

Apart from being the molecule which contains the genetic code to life, DNA also stands for 'Did Not Attend'. These three letters are often written or typed into the records of patients who fail to keep their doctors' appointment.

– NLP® –

NLP® (Neuro-Linguistic Programming) is a powerful tool that can change behaviour, aid recovery from illness and help to model success. It works through focusing on the interplay between communication (verbal and non-verbal) and its effect on emotion, performance, attitude and mental processes. Some of its roots are related to hypnotherapy, and much emphasis is placed on the power of the unconscious mind. NLP® is gradually becoming more popular in medicine, with applications to mental health, pain management and accelerated healing. It was jointly developed by Dr Richard Bandler and Professor John Grinder.

– A TYPICAL NHS HOSPITAL PATIENT LUNCH MENU –

Orange juice	Brown bread
Boiled gammon and pineapple	White bread
Cheese and tomato flan	Kosher/Halal options
Pilchard	Apple crumble
Side salad	Custard
Mixed vegetables	Tapioca pudding
Pasta salad	Jelly and ice cream
Brown rice	Apple
Boiled potatoes	

– REFLEXOLOGY –

Reflexology is an ancient system of deep massage on reflex points of the feet or hands to prevent, diagnose and treat disease anywhere in the body. Each reflex point correlates to an organ or body part. The technique was being used in both Egypt and China some 5000 years ago.

– COUNTRIES WITH THE LONGEST LIFE EXPECTANCY IN RANK ORDER –

1. Japan
2. Sweden
3. Canada
4. France
5. Australia
6. Spain
7. Finland
8. Netherlands
9. UK
10. Denmark
11. Belgium
12. USA
13. Germany

– BLOOD GROUP COMPATIBILITY –

Patient's Blood Group	Antigen on Red Cells	Antibody in Serum	Whole Blood	Red Blood Cell	Plasma
O	No A or B	Anti-A Anti-B	O	O	O, A B, AB
A	A	Anti-B	A	A, O	A, AB
B	B	Anti-A	B	B, O	B, AB
AB	A and B	None	AB	AB A, B, O	AB

– DOG BITES –

Approximately 200,000 people are bitten by dogs every year in the UK.

– SOME MILESTONES IN DRUG THERAPY DURING THE 2OTH CENTURY –

1910	Oxygen is used therapeutically for the first time
1921	Insulin is isolated in Canada
1929	Progesterone and testosterone are isolated
1937	Sulphonamides are discovered (first antibiotics)
1938	Phenytoin is introduced to treat epilepsy
1939	The insecticide DDT (dichlorodiphenyltrichloroethane) is developed and the death rate from malaria drops as a result
1940	Penicillin is used therapeutically for the first time
1943	Streptomycin is the first effective treatment for tuberculosis
1948	The antidepressant imipramine is created
1949	Cortisone is used to treat rheumatoid arthritis
1952	The polio vaccine is produced by Salk
1955	The first oral contraceptive pill is tried out in Puerto Rico
1963	Valium® (diazepam) is introduced for treating anxiety
1987	The antidepressant Prozac® (fluoxetine) is introduced
1998	Viagra® (sildenafil) is introduced to treat erectile dysfunction

– DRUG TYPES BANNED IN SPORT BY THE WORLD ANTI-DOPING AGENCY –

Stimulants	Beta-2 agonists (except in asthma)
Narcotics	Masking agents
Cannabinoids	Anabolic agents
Steroids	Diuretics
Anti-oestrogens	Peptide hormones and analogues

– SPORTS WITH IN-COMPETITION ALCOHOL (ETHANOL) PROHIBITION –

Aeronautics	Karate
Archery	Modern pentathlon
Automobile	Motorcycling
Billiards	Roller sports
Boules	Skiing
Football	Triathlon
Gymnastics	Wrestling

– SOME AMERICAN AND BRITISH MEDICAL TERMS COMPARED –

American	British
Operating room (OR)	Operating theatre
Emergency room (ER)	Accident and Emergency (A&E)
Epinephrine	Adrenaline
Acetaminophen	Paracetamol
History and physical	History and examination
Family Practice	General Practice
Attending Physician	Consultant
Chem. seven	Liver function tests (LFT)
Complete blood count (CBC)	Full blood count (FBC)

– CHARACTERISTICS OF PAIN –

Site

Radiation

Intensity

Duration

Onset (sudden or gradual)

Character (sharp, dull, colicky, etc.)

Associated features (nausea, etc.)

Exacerbating factors

Relieving factors

– BENEFITS OF BREASTFEEDING –

Breast-fed babies are less likely to have the following:

Ear infections	Diarrhoea
Allergies	Pneumonia
Vomiting	Meningitis

Breast milk:
Is easier to digest
Needs no preparation
Costs nothing
Is good for the environment

A mother who breast feeds:
Burns more calories
Can reduce her risk of ovarian cancer and breast cancer
Strengthens her bones
Helps the uterus return to its normal size

– A RANDOM POEM ABOUT GOD AND THE DOCTOR –

God and the doctor we like adore,

But only when in danger, not before;

The danger o'er, both are like requited,

God is forgotten, and the doctor slighted.

John Owen, c 1620

– A LIST OF ANTIMALARIAL MEDICINES AVAILABLE IN THE UK –

Atovaquone plus proguanil
Doxycycline
Proguanil
Mefloquine
Chloroquine
Artemether
Lumefantrine

– BLOOD PRESSURE –

In 95% of cases, the cause of high blood pressure is unknown. High blood pressure is also called 'hypertension' and is a condition that can run in families. Most people are unable to tell if they have high blood pressure. This is because most of the time it is impossible to see or to feel. Some people may experience headaches, blurred vision or tiredness.

It is a major cause of heart disease and strokes, and can cause kidney failure and blindness if left untreated long term.

High blood pressure is undertreated, with one study showing that a half of all sufferers do not have their pressure adequately controlled.

'White coat' hypertension is a term used for raised blood pressure caused by a visit to a doctor.

– TOMATOES AND LYCOPENES –

Lycopenes are members of a group of chemical compounds called carotenoids with powerful antioxidant properties that can decrease the risk of cancer and heart disease. Most of the evidence for this has been shown through work on prostate cancer, where the growth of cancer cells has been inhibited by the lycopenes found in tomatoes.

Tomato sauces, ketchup, puree and the canned variety all contain high levels of lycopenes, while tomato juice has a slightly lower concentration. This is because lycopenes are particularly concentrated in the skin of tomatoes.

– NORWALK VIRUS –

Norwalk virus was identified after an outbreak of a gastrointestinal illness in 1972 in Norwalk, Ohio. It is spread by faeces and is found in salads and shellfish (particularly oysters). Outbreaks can occur anywhere, but are more common on cruise ships and in hotels. On occasion the dumping of sewage near trawlers is to blame. The illness causes vomiting and diarrhoea.

– THE GENERAL MEDICAL COUNCIL'S 'DUTIES OF A DOCTOR' –

In particular, as a doctor you must:

Make the care of your patient your first concern;

Treat every patient politely and considerately;

Respect patients' dignity and privacy;

Listen to patients and respect their views;

Give patients information in a way they can understand;

Respect the rights of patients to be fully involved in decisions about their care;

Keep your professional knowledge and skills up to date;

Recognize the limits of your professional competence;

Be honest and trustworthy;

Respect and protect confidential information;

Make sure that your personal beliefs do not prejudice your patients' care;

Act quickly to protect patients from risk if you have good reason to believe that you or a colleague may not be fit to practise;

Avoid abusing your position as a doctor;

Work with colleagues in the ways that best serve patients' interests.

– GROUP B STREPTOCOCCUS –

Group B 'strep', as it is commonly referred to, is a bacterium that is carried by about 25% of all women. It is only really of any consequence during pregnancy. Rarely, the baby can develop infection after birth, but precautions during labour can prevent this. Approximately 98% of babies born to infected mothers will not develop infection, as long as the mother is treated. Maternal infection is detected by vaginal swabs during pregnancy.

– TATT –

Approximately 2% of patients who go to see their GP or family doctor, complain of being 'tired all the time' (TATT). In 75% of cases there are symptoms of emotional distress. About 10% of cases have a physical cause.

– SOME COMMON SECTIONS OF THE MENTAL HEALTH ACT (1983) RELATING TO MENTAL DISORDERS –

Section	Reason for admission	Legal requirements	Duration
2	Assessment	Two medical recommendations	Up to 28 days
3	Treatment	Two medical recommendations	Up to 6 months
4	Emergency	One medical recommendation	Up to 72 hours
5(2)	Doctors' power to hold inpatients	Written report to managers	Up to 72 hours
5(4)	Nurses' power to hold inpatient	Written report to managers	Up to 6 hours
135	Police warrant to remove patients	Police only	Up to 72 hours
136	Police power over mentally disordered persons in public places	Police only	Up to 72 hours

– HOW TO STOP A NEWBORN BABY FROM CRYING –

Place the palm of the hand gently over the baby's chest and abdomen and match its breathing movements for a few seconds. This usually settles babies under a week of age almost immediately on most occasions.

– DEATHS THAT MUST BE REPORTED TO THE CORONER OR THE PROCURATOR FISCAL IN THE UK –

A sudden or unexpected death

Accidents and injuries causing death

Industrial diseases

Service disability pensioners

Unknown cause of death

Deaths where the doctor has not attended within 14 days

Deaths resulting from neglect, starvation or hypothermia

Deaths in hospital within 24 hours of admission

Poisoning

Medical mishaps

Terminations

Prisoners

Stillbirths (if any doubt whether the baby was born alive)

– DYSDIADOCHOKINESIS –

Dysdiadochokinesis is the loss of ability to perform rapid repetitive movements such as touching the back of one hand with the other and then touching the palms together repeatedly as quickly as possible. This happens when a part of the brain called the cerebellum is affected, usually by a stroke or a tumour.

– SOME THINGS THAT CAN BE DETECTED BY URINE DIPSTICK TESTS –

Reagent strips can test for the following in the urine:

Leucocytes	Specific gravity
Protein	Ketones
pH	Bilirubin
Blood	Urobilinogen
Nitrites	Glucose

– ADULT NORMAL VALUES –

Haematology

Haemoglobin	Men: 13–18 g/dL
	Women: 11.5–16 g/dL
Mean cell volume	76–96 fL
Platelets	150–400 x 10^9/L
White cells (total)	4–11 x 10^9/L
Neutrophils	40–75%
Lymphocytes	20–45%
Eosinophils	1–6%
Blood gases (kPa)	PaO_2 > 10.6, $PaCO_2$ 4.7 – 6
Blood pH	7.35–7.45

Urea and electrolytes (U&E)

Sodium	135–145 mmol/L
Potassium	3.5–5 mmol/L
Creatinine	70–150 µmol/L
Urea	2.5–6.7 mmol/L
Calcium	2.12–2.65 mmol/L
Albumin	35–50 g/L
Proteins	60–80 g/L

Liver function tests (LFT)

Bilirubin	3–17 µmol/L
Alanine aminotransferase (ALT)	3–35 iu/L
Aspartate aminotransferase (AST)	3–35 iu/L
Alkaline phosphatase (ALP)	30–300 iu/L

Some other tests

Prostate-specific antigen (PSA)	0–4 ng/mL
	(age-dependent)
Thyroxine (T_4)	70–140 mmol/L
Thyroid-stimulating hormone (TSH)	0.5–5 mu/L
Fasting glucose	3.0–6.0 mmol/L
C-reactive protein (CRP)	<10 mg/L

– HEMISPHERIC DOMINANCE –

99% of right-handed people have a dominant left cerebral hemisphere, whereas only 40% of left handers have a dominant right cerebral hemisphere.

– A LOOK AT THE NAILS –

Nail feature and description	What it might suggest
Koilonychia (spoon-shaped nails)	Iron deficiency, syphilis, heart disease
Onycholysis (destruction of nails)	Hyperthyroidism, fungal nail infection, psoriasis
Beau's lines (transverse furrows across all nails, which occur if nail growth stops)	A recent severe illness
Mees' lines (paired parallel transverse lines)	Low albumin
Terry's lines (white nails with pink tips)	Liver cirrhosis
Pitting (tiny dimples on the nail surface)	Psoriasis or alopecia areata
Splinter haemorrhages (long streaks of dark red haemorrhages)	Endocarditis or trauma to the nail
Clubbing (the nails look excessively curved in length, giving the finger a drumstick appearance)	Can be harmless if born with it (i.e. congenital); lung cancer, cystic fibrosis, Crohn's disease, cirrhosis, a gut lymphoma, endocarditis, congenital heart disease

– SOME FAMOUS PSYCHOANALYSTS –

Sigmund Freud (1856–1939)
Carl Jung (1875–1961)
Melanie Klein (1882–1960)
Donald Winnicott (1897–1971)

– TAKING BLOOD (VENEPUNCTURE) –

1. Set out the necessary equipment, which includes a tourniquet, rubber gloves, a piece of cotton wool, a sterile alcohol wipe, a plaster, the relevant blood bottles to be filled, a green needle and a syringe (which will be described below) or, as is now preferred, a Vacutainer® and its needle.
2. Tell the patient what is about to happen.
3. Put on the rubber gloves.
4. Find an obvious vein in the antecubital fossa (in between the forearm and the upper arm) – they will have a green tinge.
5. Confirm the vein by feeling it – it should feel slightly rubbery.
6. Place and tie the tourniquet above the vein (proximal to it).
7. Wipe the vein with the alcohol wipe.
8. If the patient is nervous, reassure and distract. If there is any possibility of fainting, lie him or her down.
9. Place the needle on the end of the syringe and advance the needle into the vein carefully.
10. Once the vein has been pierced, a flashback of blood fills the green part of the needle.
11. After this, slowly draw back the plunger of the syringe, which will fill with blood.
12. Once the syringe is almost full, release the tourniquet with the free hand, and withdraw the needle, taking care to be quick about applying pressure to the puncture site with cotton wool (the patient may take over applying this pressure).
13. Carefully puncture the tops of each blood bottle with the needle, and the blood will quickly flow into them.
14. Discard the syringe and needle immediately into a sharps bin.
15. Replace the cotton wool with a plaster and ensure that the patient is all right.

– THE HEART AND ITS STRENGTH –

The heart beats approximately 72 times per minute, pushing 5 litres of blood around the circulation in that time. The heart beats about 4 million times a year and 3 billion times in an average Western lifespan.

– PATIENTS' PHRASES COMMONLY HEARD BY GENERAL PRACTITIONERS –

'I'm not worried about it, but my wife forced me to come and see you ...'

'I think I need something strong to shift this ...'

'I've got a really stressful job ...'

'I've had a cough for about six weeks now and I just can't seem to shift it ...'

'While I'm here ...'

'Can you speed up my hospital appointment please?'

'I didn't want to take painkillers in case I did more damage to myself ...'

'I think it's time I had a scan or something ...'

'I'm tired all the time ...'

'Work want a sick note ...'

'I don't come very often, so I've saved up quite a few things ...'

'What are you going to do about my drink problem?'

'Yes, but ...'

'I think I'm just really run down ...'

'I can't swallow tablets ...'

'I've always smoked ...'

'You're running a bit late this evening ...'

– PHRENOLOGY –

Phrenology is an ancient practice that became particularly popular during Victorian times. It involves the study of the shape and form of the skull and its relation to character, emotions and intellectual capacity. Phrenologists can map out areas such as spirituality and benevolence across different parts of the brain.

– POINTS TO NOTE DURING A NEONATAL EXAMINATION (USUALLY BETWEEN 24 AND 48 HOURS AFTER BIRTH) –

General appearance
Jaundice
Cyanosis
Pallor
Syndrome features
Birthmarks
Lanugo

Head and facial features
Head circumference
Cephalohaematoma
Fontanelles
Accessory auricles
Red reflex
Hare lip
Jaw
Cleft lip or palate
Ebstein's pearls
Low-set ears

Upper limb
Webbing of fingers
Palmar creases
Number of fingers
Erb's palsy
Normal movements

Cardiovascular system
Femoral pulses
Heart sounds and murmurs

Abdomen
Umbilical hernia
Umbilical cord
Umbilical infection
Masses

Nervous system
Normal Moro reflex
Head movement
Limb movement
Normal cry

Back
Sacral pit
Spina bifida
Scoliosis

Hips
Barlow's and
Ortolani's tests

Lower limb
Skin creases
Femoral pulses
Talipes

Genitalia
Penis shape
Hypospadias
Hernia
Testes
Hydrocele
Vaginal tag
Bleeding

– HOW TO TAKE BLOOD PRESSURE MANUALLY –

1. Either arm will do, although conventionally the right arm is chosen
2. Place the cuff around the patient's upper arm
3. Locate the patient's radial pulse in the same arm
4. Place a stethoscope in your ears
5. Place the stethoscope over the brachial artery, just below the cuff
6. Inflate the cuff while feeling the radial pulse (at the wrist). It will 'disappear' at some point, as will any sound through the stethoscope.
7. Once this happens, start to *slowly* deflate the cuff and watch the numbers on the gauge attached to the cuff
8. When the first sound appears, this is the *systolic* pressure
9. When the last sound disappears, this is the *diastolic* pressure
10. The blood pressure is the *systolic/diastolic* pressure and is expressed in mmHg (millimetres of mercury)

– SOME INTERNAL ORGANS AND STRUCTURES WITHOUT WHICH WE CAN SURVIVE UNAIDED –

One kidney	Prostate
Gallbladder	Uterus
Appendix	Veins (e.g. varicose)

– IQ RANGES –

Above 130	Very superior intelligence
121 – 130	Superior intelligence
111 – 120	High average intelligence
100 – 110	Average intelligence
70 – 99	Borderline mental retardation
50 – 69	Mild mental retardation
35 – 49	Moderate mental retardation
20 – 34	Severe mental retardation
Below 20	Profound mental retardation

– SOME MEDICAL CONDITIONS THAT NEED TO BE NOTIFIED TO THE UK DVLA (DRIVER AND VEHICLE LICENSING AGENCY) –

Epilepsy
Fits and blackouts
Severe and recurrent giddiness
Parkinson's disease
Multiple sclerosis
Motor neurone disease
Stroke
Brain tumour or surgery
Severe head injury
Serious memory problems
Narcolepsy and cataplexy
Mental health conditions
Cardiovascular disorders

Visual disorders
Diabetes mellitus
Any heart condition
Certain cancers
Spinal injuries
Renal disorders
Respiratory and sleep disorders
Impaired limb function or
    amputation
Behavioural problems
Any other medical
    condition likely to affect
    driving ability

– CAESAREAN SECTION –

Caesarean section is a surgical procedure that is becoming increasingly common in the UK and takes its name from the fact that Julius Caesar was apparently born by this method in 100 BC. That this actually happened is highly unlikely, bearing in mind that there were no antibiotics, and that Caesar's mother survived the procedure – a near impossibility in those times. In fact, in ancient times, the procedure was usually performed in the event of maternal death.

– AMOK –

Amok was first described among Malay warriors in the 16th century. It is exclusive to men and is characterized by sudden homicidal behaviour. The sufferer (pengamok) is usually triggered by insults and will only stop his behaviour if overcome or killed by others. Some experts hypothesize that restrictions in the adolescent period can lead to this behaviour. Others think that a major life event may be the trigger. Unsurprisingly, the phrase to 'run amok' is derived from this condition.

– THE CHILDHOOD VACCINE SCHEDULE (UK) –

Vaccine	Age when given
BCG	Birth or 10–14 years
Diphtheria Tetanus Pertussis Hib Meningitis C Polio	2 months (1st dose) 3 months (2nd dose) 4 months (3rd dose)
(MMR) Measles Mumps Rubella	13 months
Pre-school booster of: Diphtheria Tetanus Pertussis Polio MMR	3–5 years
Leaving school booster of: Tetanus Diphtheria Polio	13–18 years

Hepatitis B (only to
    children of high-risk
    mothers or mothers
    with Hep B infection)
	Birth
	1 month
	2 months
	12-month booster

– SOME MEDICAL CONDITIONS AND NAMES CONTAINING COLOURS –

Yellow fever	Black death
Blue naevus	Red reflex
Grey man syndrome	White cells
Scarlet fever	

– SENSATE FOCUS FOR SEXUAL DYSFUNCTION (MASTERS & JOHNSON, 1970) –

Stage one	Touching partner without genital contact for subject's own pleasure
Stage two	Touching partner without genital contact for subject's and partner's pleasure
Stage three	Touching partner with genital contact, but intercourse not permitted
Stage four	Simultaneous touching of partner and being touched by partner with genital contact, but intercourse not permitted
Stage five	If both feel ready, the female invites the male to put his penis into her vagina. Female on top position heightens female control and allows male to relax. No thrusting. Initial containment brief, lengthening period of containment with each session.
Stage six	Vaginal containment with movement. Different positions are encouraged. Does not inevitably lead to climax. Couple practise stopping before climax. Provided physical contact is pleasurable, orgasm is not necessary.

(Masters WH, Johnson VE (1970) *Human Sexual Inadequacy*. London, Churchill)

– SKIN –

The skin is the body's largest 'organ'. It makes up about 15% of body weight and has a surface area of around 2 square metres in an adult.

– PREGNANCY TESTS –

Both blood and urinary pregnancy tests pick up the presence of human chorionic gonadotrophin (hCG). These tests are 98% accurate for a positive result.

– BARTHEL ACTIVITIES OF DAILY LIVING INDEX –

Bowels
0 – incontinent, needs enemas
1 – occasional accident
2 – continent

Bladder
0 – incontinent or catheterized, unable to manage alone
1 – occasional accident
2 – continent

Grooming
0 – needs help with personal care
1 – independent face/teeth/hair/shaving

Toilet use
0 – dependent
1 – needs some help, but can do something
2 – independent; can get on and off and is able to dress/wipe

Stairs
0 – unable
1 – needs help
2 – independent

Bathing
0 – dependent
1 – independent

Transfer (bed to chair and back)
0 – Unable, no sitting balance
1 – major help (one or two people), sits
2 – minor help
3 – independent

Mobility
0 – immobile
1 – wheelchair-dependent
2 – walks with help of one person
3 – independent (may have stick, etc.

Dressing
0 – dependent
1 – needs help, can do half unaided
2 – independent (including buttons, zips, etc.)

Score
<15 usually represents moderate disability
< 10 usually represents severe disability

(Mahoney FI, Barthel DW, Functional evaluation: the Barthel Index. *Maryland State Medical Journal*, February 1965, vol 14, 56. Used with permission)

– URINARY CATHETERS –

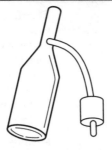

Urinary catheters are used during operations as well as on a permanent basis by some people. There are two systems by which catheters are sized: the Gauge sizing system and the French sizing system.

The approximate outside diameter in millimeters can be calculated by dividing the French (Fr) size by 3. For example, a 12 Fr catheter has an outside diameter of 4 mm. The French system is logical: the bigger the number, the bigger the catheter (the largest being 30 Fr). The Gauge system is inverse: the bigger the number, the smaller the catheter.

Once the catheter has been inserted into the bladder through the urethra, a balloon is inflated around the catheter tube inside the bladder to stop it from slipping down and out of the bladder.

– THE COST OF SOME PRIVATE OPERATIONS IN THE UK (£) –

Procedure	Cost (£)
Cataract removal	1250–2800
Heart bypass	11,000–15,000
Hernia treatment	1400–2000
Hip replacement	6000–12,000
Hysterectomy	3000–5700
Knee replacement	8000–11,000
Varicose vein treatment	1400–2000
Vasectomy	150–1200

– A JOKE TOLD TO A PSYCHIATRIST BY ONE OF HER PATIENTS –

'What's the difference between a psychiatrist and a terrorist?'
'You can negotiate with a terrorist.'

– MEDICAL EPONYMS STARTING WITH EACH LETTER OF THE ALPHABET –

Addison's disease
Bell's palsy
Campbell de Morgan spot
Dupytren's contracture
Ehlers-Danlos syndrome
Felty's syndrome
Graves' disease
Huntington's chorea
Ice skater's fracture
Jakob-Creutzfeld disease
Kaposi's sarcoma
Laurence-Biedl-Moon syndrome
Munchausen's syndrome
Nelson's syndrome

Osgood-Schlatter disease
Peyronie's disease
Quincke's oedema
Raynaud's syndrome
Steel-Richardson-Olszewski
  syndrome
Tietze's syndrome
Uhthoff's sign
Virchow's node
Wegener's granulomatosis
XX Turner phenotype
  syndrome
Yankauer sucker
Zollinger-Ellison syndrome

– HOW MUCH CAN YOUR BLADDER HOLD? –

The capacity of the adult bladder varies from 400 ml to 800 ml. The desire to pass urine can start at 200 ml content, but can be controlled by signals from the brain.

– NOTIFIABLE INDUSTRIAL DISEASES –

Poisoning by industrial agents
Repetitive strain injury
Vibration white finger
Bursitis
Occupational asthma
Occupational infection

Chrome ulceration
Irritant dermatitis
Pneumoconiosis
Extrinsic allergic alveolitis
Occupational deafness
Occupational cancers

– SOME THINGS TO AVOID IN PREGNANCY –

Smoking
Alcohol
Vitamin A supplements
Liver
Uncooked eggs
Undercooked food, especially
  meat
Pâté
Cat faeces
Flying after 36 weeks of
  pregnancy
Rubella
Lambing season
Peanuts

– THE HUMAN GENOME PROJECT –

The Human Genome Project began in 1990 in the USA and was a large international project dedicated to identify all the genes in human DNA *(qv)*. It was completed in 2003 and the information gathered is likely to have profound effects on the way in which diseases are detected and treated, in addition to methods of assessing health risks, identifying victims or perpetrators of crime, developing vaccines and providing many more benefits to mankind.

– JOHN MILTON ON HIS BLINDNESS –

When I consider how my light is spent
Ere half my days in this dark world and wide,
And that one talent which is death to hide
Lodged with me useless, though my soul more bent
To serve therewith my Maker, and present
My true account, lest he returning chide,
'Doth God exact day-labor, light denied?'
I fondly ask! But Patience, to prevent
That murmur, soon replies: 'God doth not need
Either man's work or his own gifts; who best
Bear his mild yoke, they serve him best. His state
Is kingly: thousands at his bidding speed
And post o'er land and ocean without rest;
They also serve who also stand and wait.'

John Milton, 1608–1674

– THE COST OF TRAINING A DOCTOR IN THE UK –

The cost of training a doctor in the UK is approximately £250,000.

– HIV AND AIDS –

In the last year almost 5 million people became infected with HIV worldwide, according to statistics released by UNAIDS. Interestingly, there has been a sharp rise in the number of young women with the disease and this group is now in the high-risk category. Nearly half of all people infected with HIV are now women and almost 40 million people worldwide are now estimated to be living with HIV. The quest for a vaccine is looking promising at the time of writing.

– ECG –

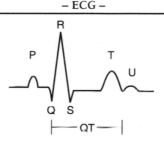

The ECG (electrocardiogram) was invented by Wilhelm Einthoven, a Dutch physiologist, in 1895. He was awarded the Nobel prize for his creation in 1924. The ECG is a common investigation, which shows the electrical activity of the heart and thus reveals any defect in the workings of the heart's muscle. It is used to confirm heart attacks, heart failure and gives characteristic appearances in a patient with pulmonary embolus or certain chemical imbalances. It is also used routinely in some patients before surgery. Each beat of the heart is displayed by waves, which are given letters. These include P, Q, R, S, T, J and U waves. There are also delta waves.

– THE HEIMLICH MANOEUVRE (FOR CHOKING) –

A choking victim can't speak or breathe and needs your help immediately. Follow these steps to help a choking victim:

From behind, wrap your arms around the victim's waist.

Make a fist and place the thumb side of your fist against the victim's upper abdomen, below the ribcage and above the navel.

Grasp your fist with your other hand and press into their upper abdomen with a quick upward thrust. Do not squeeze the ribcage; confine the force of the thrust to your hands.

Repeat until the object is expelled.

The Heimlich manoeuvre was invented in 1974 by Dr Henry Heimlich, who now presides over the Heimlich Institute. There are variations of the manoeuvre for drowning and asthma and for performing it on oneself. Carrie Fisher, Elizabeth Taylor, Goldie Hawn, Ronald Reagan, Walter Matthau, Jack Lemmon and Cher have all been saved by this famous manouevre.

– TYPES OF SHOCK –

Hypovolaemic	Septic
Cardiogenic	Neurogenic

– SOME FEMALE FACTS –

Among Western nations, the Netherlands has the lowest incidence of teenage pregnancy and abortion

The first vibrator was invented in 1869 and was powered by steam. It was used to treat 'female disorders'

In the late 1800s vulval massage used to be a treatment for hysteria and sulphuric acid was used to treat nymphomania

Women are much more likely to commit adultery when they are ovulating

During foreplay, a woman's breasts can increase in size by up to 25%

The average female orgasm lasts about 50 seconds

– BEETHOVEN AND HEARING –

Ludwig van Beethoven (1770–1827), was one of the greatest ever composers. At the age of 31 he started to lose his hearing, and by the age of 50 he was totally deaf. His last symphony (Symphony No. 9) was the first of its kind to have a chorus and was received with a standing ovation. Ironically, he was unable to hear the work himself. He is likely to have suffered from otosclerosis, a condition caused by stiffening and overgrowth of bone in the ear.

– ON WALKING –

In an average lifetime a person walks about 70,000 miles – more than twice the world's circumference.

– SEEING A 'SHRINK' –

The term 'shrink' used colloquially to refer to a psychiatrist is from the slang American term 'headshrinker', which was first coined in the 1950s.

– MOZART'S CAUSE OF DEATH –

After the death of the great composer Wolfgang Amadeus Mozart, there was much speculation about whether he had been poisoned by his rival Antonio Salieri. Doctors working with a Mozart scholar at the University of Maryland School of Medicine recently concluded that Mozart died of rheumatic fever. This was a common ailment at the time but is much rarer today because of the existence and use of antibiotics.

– THE COST OF CHOLESTEROL-BUSTING –

In the UK the average cost per person per year, to whomever is paying, of being on a statin to lower cholesterol is £150–£650, depending on the dose.

– SOME FACTS RELATED TO MALE GENITALIA –

The odours of lavender, liquorice and chocolate supposedly increase blood flow to the penis

The word 'penis' is derived from the Latin word meaning 'tail'

The left testicle usually hangs lower than the right, although the reverse may be true of left-handed men

Sperm have to swim 100,000 times their length in order to get a woman pregnant

Approximately 22% of British men are circumcised

The average male orgasm lasts about 13 seconds

The average condom is 0.07 mm thick

– HOW A GENERAL PRACTITIONER MIGHT CONDUCT A CONSULTATION WITH A PATIENT –

Find out why the patient has attended

Address the patient's ideas, concerns and expectations

Consider other ongoing problems

Choose an appropriate action for each problem

Achieve a shared understanding with the patient

Involve the patient in the management plan

Use time and resources appropriately

Maintain a good relationship with the patient

– TRUANCY –

Truancy is the intentional avoidance of school. It is often accompanied by antisocial behaviour, is more likely to happen in a large family and is linked with poor performance at school. This is different from when a child refuses to go to school (school refusal) – which is usually related to anxiety.

– HOW A HOSPITAL DOCTOR MIGHT CONDUCT A CONSULTATION WITH A PATIENT –

Presenting complaint
History of presenting complaint
Past medical and surgical history
Drug history and allergies
Social history
Examination
Investigations
Management plan and definitive care

– FOUR TYPES OF 'HEARTSINK' PATIENTS (GROVES, 1978) –

Dependent clinger
Entitled demander
Manipulative help rejecter
Self-destructive denier

(Groves JE, Taking care of the hateful patient. *New England Journal of Medicine*, April 1978, vol 298, 883)

– NUTRITION FROM WHITE BREAD (per 100 g) –

Energy 986 kJ/230 kcal	Fat 2.2 g
Protein 8.2 g	Fibre 2.8 g
Carbohydrate 44.1 g	Sodium 0.5 g

– SOFT DRINKS AND SOME POWERFUL ADDITIVES –

Amazingly, Coca-Cola® originally used to contain small amounts of cocaine. This was in the days when cocaine was as freely available as aspirin at the local shop. It was developed from a drink called the 'French wine of Coca'. The drink 7-UP® originally contained lithium, which of course is a potent drug used as a mood stabilizer or to treat manic depression.

– SOME UNOFFICIAL MEDICAL SLANG –

RATTFO . . . . Reassured and told to fuck off
Acopia . . . . Patient attending for help who is unable to cope
Orthopod . . . . An orthopaedic surgeon
10 and 2 . . . . 10 mg haloperidol and 2 mg lorazepam (in emergency)
Gerifix . . . . A cocktail of an antibiotic and a diuretic to treat the elderly
FLK . . . . Funny-looking kid
Cheese and Onion . . The *Oxford Handbook of Clinical Medicine*
Went off . . . . (A patient) suddenly deteriorated

– SLEEP –

In general, the older we get, the less sleep we need.

– ANTHRAX –

Anthrax is an infectious disease caused by *Bacillus anthracis*, which forms spores. It occurs most commonly in cattle but it can occur in humans when they are exposed to infected animals, or to spores from their remains. There are three ways in which anthrax can infect humans: through inhalation, through the intestine and through the skin. The inhalation route causes almost certain death, and bioterrorists kill people by posting spores in envelopes to innocent recipients.

– THERMOMETER –

The first thermometer was water-based and invented by Galileo Galilei in 1593.

– GIVING BLOOD –

In Paraguay, duelling is legal provided both parties are registered blood donors.

– OCCUPATIONAL CLASSIFICATION BY THE UK OFFICE OF POPULATION, CENSUSES AND SURVEYS (OPCS) –

I	Professionals, landowners
II	Intermediate
III	Skilled manual, clerical
IV	Semi-skilled
V	Unskilled
0	Students, unemployed

– LAYERS OF THE SCALP –

Skin
    Connective tissue
        Aponeurosis
            Loose areolar tissue
                Pericranium

– SILENT GENIUS –

Albert Einstein did not speak until the age of six years.

– RING FINGER –

In ancient Egypt it was believed that there was a nerve connecting the fourth finger of the left hand to the heart – hence it became used for the wearing of wedding bands.

– BRANCHES OF THE TRIGEMINAL NERVE –

Ophthalmic division – nasociliary, frontal and lacrimal nerves

Maxillary division – infraorbital, zygomaticofacial and zygomaticotemporal nerves

Mandibular division – buccal, auriculotemporal, inferior alv
and lingual nerves

– SOME SIGNS TO LOOK FOR IN THE HANDS (EXCLUDING THE NAILS) –

Sign	Possible diagnosis
Palmar erythema	Liver cirrhosis, pregnancy, polycythaemia
Dupuytren's contracture	Liver disease, trauma, ageing
Pigmented creases	Addison's disease
Heberden's nodes	Osteoarthritis
Osler's nodes	Endocarditis

– THE 12 CRANIAL NERVES –

I	Olfactory	VII	Facial
II	Optic	VIII	Vestibulocochlear
III	Oculomotor	IX	Glossopharyngeal
IV	Trochlear	X	Vagus
V	Trigeminal	XI	Accessory
VI	Abducens	XII	Hypoglossal

– FAMOUS PEOPLE WHO HAVE DIED FROM AIDS –

Rock Hudson
Freddie Mercury
Denholm Elliot
Liberace
Kenny Everett

Arthur Ashe
Derek Jarman
Isaac Asimov
Ofra Haza

– HOW TO PERFORM KOCHER'S METHOD FOR REDUCTION OF A DISLOCATED SHOULDER –

1. Lie the patient flat and sedate appropriately

2. Flex the elbow to 90° and slowly and very gently externally rotate the shoulder

   Slowly adduct the upper arm across the chest with the shoulder externally rotated

   ...nce adducted maximally, internally rotate the shoulder

– BUCCINATOR –

The buccinator is a muscle in the cheek that pushes food against the teeth and is used during whistling and blowing. Trumpeters often have very prominent buccinator muscles because of powerful use of them in playing their instrument.

– CONVERTING TEMPERATURE –

To convert Celsius to Fahrenheit, multiply by 1.8 and add 32
To convert Fahrenheit to Celsius, subtract 32 and divide by 1.8

– HIP CEMENT –

The cement used in hip replacements is called polymethyl methacrylate (PMMA).

– A NON-EXHAUSTIVE LIST OF SOME MEDICAL PATRON SAINTS –

AIDS patients	Aloysius Gonzaga
Alcoholics	John of God
Amputees	Anthony of Padua
Babies and infants	Brigid of Ireland
Bacterial infections	Agrippina
Birth	Erasmus
Blind	Catald
Convulsions/epilepsy	John the Baptist
Death	Christopher
Dieticians	Martha
Disabled	Giles
Doctors	Luke the Apostle
Domestic workers	Adelelmus
Elderly people	Anthony of Padua
Health	Infant Jesus of Prague
Hospitals	Camillus of Lellis
Medical record librarians	Raymond of Penyafort
Nurses	Agatha
Paramedics	Michael the Archangel
Pharmacists	Mary Magdalen

– NOBEL PRIZE WINNERS IN PHYSIOLOGY AND MEDICINE IN THE LAST DECADE –

Year	Recipient(s) and discovery
1994	Alfred Gilman and Martin Rodbell, regarding G-proteins and the role of these proteins in signal transduction in cells
1995	Edward Lewis, Christiane Nüsslein-Volhard and Eric Wieschaus, regarding the genetic control of early embryonic development
1996	Peter Doherty and Rolf Zinkernagel, regarding the specificity of the cell-mediated immune defence
1997	Stanley Prusiner, regarding prions
1998	Robert Furchgott, Louis Ignarro and Ferid Murad, regarding nitric oxide as a signalling molecule in the cardiovascular system.
1999	Günter Blobel, regarding protein signalling that governs transport and localization in the cell.
2000	Arvid Carlsson, Paul Greengard and Eric Kandel, regarding signal transduction in the nervous system
2001	Leland Hartwell, R Timothy Hunt and Paul Nurse, regarding key regulators of the cell cycle
2002	Sydney Brenner, H Robert Horvitz and John Sulston, regarding genetic regulation of organ development and programmed cell death
2003	Sir Peter Mansfield and Paul Lauterbur, regarding magnetic resonance imaging
2004	Richard Axel and Linda B Buck, regarding discoveries of odorant receptors and the organization of the olfactory system

– THE STAGES OF GRIEF –

1. Shock
2. Sadness
3. Anger
4. Denial
5. Irritability
6. Somatic distress
7. Identification phenomena

– EBOLA –

The Ebola virus was first identified in Sudan in 1976 after epidemics both there and in Zaire. Ebola is a haemorrhagic fever – which means that the infected persons can bleed profusely. It is one of the deadliest diseases known to mankind, causing death in most cases. It is transmitted by direct contact with the blood or body fluids of infected persons or by contact with dead infected chimpanzees.

– WHO –

The World Health Organization (WHO) was set up by the United Nations in 1948. Its headquarters are in Geneva and its objective is to attain the highest possible level of health for as many people as possible. The WHO definition of health is a 'state of complete physical, mental and social well-being'.

– SOME MEDICAL SUFFIXES AND THEIR MEANINGS –

Suffix	Meaning
-ectomy	removal of
-centesis	tap or puncture
-ostomy	forming an opening
-otomy	to cut into
-pexy	fixation
-lysis	destruction
-tripsy	destruction by crushing
-algia	pain
-cele	hernia
-dynia	pain
-aemia	blood
-itis	inflammation
-megaly	enlargement
-oma	tumour
-osis	abnormal
-pathy	disease
-penia	deficiency

– THE MEDICAL PREFIXES FOR COLOURS –

Glauco- . . .	Grey	Cirrho- . . .	Yellow
Leuco-	White	Cyano- . . .	Blue
Erythro- . . .	Red	Chloro- . . .	Green
Melano- . . .	Black		

– SOME FAMOUS CIGARETTE SMOKERS –

George Harrison
Bob Marley
Jacqueline Kennedy Onassis
Graham Chapman
Humphrey Bogart

Nat 'King' Cole
Sammy Davis Jr
Walt Disney
Yul Brynner

– SOME CHEMICALS FOUND IN CIGARETTES AND THEIR EFFECTS –

Chemical	Effects
Ammonia	Used in toilet cleaner and dry-cleaning fluid
Acetone	Nail polish remover
Arsenic	Rat poison
Benzene	A petrol additive that causes cancer
Carbon monoxide	A gas that starves the body of oxygen
Cadmium	Used in batteries and oil paint and causes cancer
Formaldehyde	Used in embalming and causes cancer
Hydrogen cyanide	A poisonous gas used in gas chambers
Lead	Lowers IQ levels
Methoprene	An insecticide used to kill fleas
Nicotine	An insecticide and addictive chemical
Polonium	A radioactive element that causes cancer
·yrene	Found in insulation material
	A solid used on road surfaces
·ne	Used in embalming
·ine	Used in paint stripper

– SOME ETHNICALLY AND DEMOGRAPHICALLY PREVALENT DISEASES –

Thalassaemia – A disorder of synthesis of haemoglobin chains that is common in populations from Africa, the Mediterranean, the Middle East, India and South East Asia

Sickle cell anaemia – Sickling of red cells is most common in Africa, less common in the Mediterranean, Middle East and Indian populations

Tay-Sachs disease – A genetic disorder affecting children that has a much higher incidence in Ashkenazi Jews

Takayasu's arteritis – Arteritis of the renal arteries and aortic arch, common in Asia and the Far East

– CONTROLLED DRUGS (UK) –

Prescriptions for Controlled Drugs (e.g. morphine) must be in the prescriber's own handwriting and include:

The name and address of the patient

The form and strength of the preparation

The total quantity of the preparation, or the number of dose units in both words and figures

The dose

The words 'for dental treatment only' if issued by a dentist

– SOME CONDITIONS NAMED AFTER VOCATIONS, EVENTS AND ACTIVITIES –

Gamekeeper's thumb	Boxer's fracture
Pigeon fancier's lung	Clay shoveller's fracture
Tennis elbow	Dashboard dislocation
Housemaid's knee	Ice skater's fracture
Golfer's elbow	Horse rider's knee
Aviator's astragalus	Nursemaid's elbow

– STOMACH ACID –

Gastric acid is over 1500 times as strong as chip shop vinegar.

– THE UK NATIONAL TRIAGE SCALE FOR ACCIDENT AND EMERGENCY –

Triage category	Meaning and examples
1	*Immediate resuscitation* – Patients in need of immediate treatment for preservation of life (e.g. cardiac arrest)
2	*Very urgent* – Seriously ill or injured patients whose lives are not in immediate danger (e.g. severe chest pain)
3	*Urgent* – Patients with serious problems, but apparently stable condition (e.g. fracture of the hip)
4	*Standard* – Standard cases without immediate danger or distress (e.g. a sprained ankle)
5	*Non-urgent* – Patients whose conditions are not true accidents or emergencies (e.g. mild back pain that has been going on for two years)

– THE BRUCE PROTOCOL –

The Bruce Protocol was designed in 1963 by Dr Robert Bruce, an American cardiologist. It is still used today for assessing cardiovascular health using a graded uphill treadmill test. The test is multistage and there are incremental levels of difficulty, which change every three minutes. Interestingly, Dr Bruce found that over 60% of patients who took the test were then motivated to modify their lifestyle in order to improve their health.

– SUPER SURGEON –

ndian ophthalmologist Dr Murugappa Chennaveerappa Modi formed 610,564 operations between 1943 and 1993 – that's an age of 12,211 operations a year.

– PHINEAS GAGE –

Phineas Gage (1823–1860) was a railway foreman who was the victim of an explosive accident in which a tamping iron went through his cheek and destroyed a large part of his brain. Incredibly, he survived, but people around him noticed that his personality had changed dramatically. He also started to suffer from seizures. His case has helped scientists and doctors study and hypothesize about the role that different lobes of the brain have on personality.

– CHARING CROSS FOUR-LAYER BANDAGING –

Researchers at Charing Cross Hospital in Fulham, London demonstrated in the 1980s that venous leg ulcers could be healed by the use of four-layer pressure bandaging. Amazingly, this applied to chronic ulcers (which had not healed for many years). This pioneering treatment achieved healing rates of up to 80% in a local study. It has now been adopted internationally as a gold standard method for treating venous leg ulcers.

– DIALYSIS FOR RENAL FAILURE –

Over 20,000 people are on dialysis in the UK. The average cost of dialysis is approximately £30,000 per patient per year.

– THE NATIONAL PLATE MODEL –

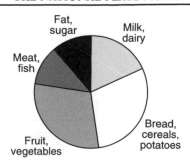

– PLACEBO FOR SALE –

Since Autumn 2003, placebo tablets (Sucrosa® by AstraZeneca) have been on sale in the USA. This type of tablet has no active ingredient, but has been shown in trials to relieve and subjectively improve symptoms such as erectile dysfunction, anxiety and pain. This is in keeping with previous studies involving the power of the mind related to physical health. People who look forward to a vaccine, for example, have been shown to mount a stronger immune response than those who don't.

– HOW DO MAGIC MUSHROOMS WORK? –

The primary active ingredients of *Psilocybe* or 'magic' mushrooms are psilocybin and psilocin. When the mushrooms are eaten, psilocybin is thought to be converted into psilocin. This is then absorbed into the blood stream, where it is taken to the brain.

Psilocin is similar in structure to serotonin (5-hydroxytryptamine, 5-HT) – a naturally occurring neurotransmitter. As such, psilocin is thought to be a 5-HT agonist – i.e. it acts on and is taken up by 5-HT receptor sites – namely 5-HT_2. LSD is thought to act in the same way. A change in 5-HT levels will affect mood, sleep, appetite and sensory perception – hence the effects felt from taking magic mushrooms, which include hallucinations, often with altered sight, taste, touch and sounds.

– SOME IRON PREPARATIONS –

Ferrous sulphate	Sodium ferdetate
Ferrous fumarate	Iron dextran
Ferrous gluconate	Iron sorbitol
Ferrous glycine sulphate	Iron sucrose
Polysaccharide-iron complex	

– NICOTINE –

...tine is named after Jean Nicot, who introduced tobacco to

– THE QUEEN'S HOSPITAL –

Her Majesty the Queen and the Royal Family are usually admitted for treatment to the King Edward VII's Hospital in Central London. 'HM Medical Household' is a select list of doctors who provide medical care to the Royal Family, forming part of 'HM Royal Household'. This household list includes doctors from general practice as well as many specialties, and is headed by a London-based consultant physician, Sir Richard Thompson.

– FIRST FEMALE DOCTOR IN ENGLAND –

The first female doctor in England was 'James' Miranda Barry, honoured for services during the Battle of Waterloo. Dr Barry had to disguise herself as a man all her life in order to study and practise medicine.

– HELMAN'S FOLK MODEL OF ILLNESS –

What has happened?

Why has it happened?

Why to me?

Why now?

What would happen if nothing were done about it?

What should I do and who should I see for further help?

(Helman CG, Disease versus illness in general practice. *Journal of the Royal College of General Practitioners*, September 1981, vol 31, 548)

– SOME DOCTOR AUTHORS –

Somerset Maugham	Sir Arthur Conan Doyle
Anton Chekhov	A J Cronin
John Keats	Gordon Ostler (Richard Gordon)

– QUARANTINE –

Quarantine comes from the Italian *quarantina*, which mea~ referring to the number of days of isolation.

– MIGRAINE –

The word 'migraine' originates from the French word *hemi-crain* 'half head'.

– FROM TESTICLES TO TESTIMONY –

The word 'testimony' is directly related to the word 'testicle'. This dates back to Roman times, when only men were allowed to give evidence and had to prove their sex by revealing their testicles to the judge. A modern equivalent of this ritual is the chromosome test that is performed by the Olympic Games Committee to prevent countries substituting a man for a woman and vice versa (a feat incredibly pulled off just a few years ago).

– GENERAL ANAESTHETIC –

Ether was the first general anaesthetic and was pioneered in the USA in the 1842 by Dr Crawford Long.

– INDIA AND HER CONTRIBUTIONS TO MEDICINE –

Approximately 38% of doctors in the USA are Indian

Sushruta, an Ayurvedic doctor from 2600 years ago, is considered by some to be a founding father of surgery

India is the world's largest and oldest continuous civilization

The Ayurveda is the oldest system of medicine known to man

– SOME CAUSES OF A RED EYE –

Conjunctivitis	Blepharitis
Orbital cellulitis	Foreign body
Episcleritis	Acute glaucoma
Scleritis	Corneal ulceration
Subconjunctival haemorrhage	Dacrocystitis

– SOME CONDITIONS THAT MAY WARRANT A STOMA –

Carcinoma

Diverticula

Bowel ischaemia

Trauma

Hirschsprung's disease

Obstruction

Crohn's disease

Faecal incontinence

Ulcerative colitis

Familial polyposis coli

Radiotherapy

Meconium ileus

Fistula

– PERCUSSION AND BEER –

Percussion is part of the four-stage process that doctors use to examine patients. Inspection (looking) is first; palpation (feeling) is next, followed by percussion (tapping) and then auscultation (listening). It involves tapping, for instance on the lungs to reveal whether the lung has any fluid in it. A dull sound suggests fluid, whereas a resonant sound usually suggests air. It was first noticed by a physician who saw a brewer banging his barrels of beer with a stick to work out how full they were.

– BASIC LIFE SUPPORT –

CHECK RESPONSIVENESS – *if no response,*
SHOUT FOR HELP
OPEN AIRWAY
CHECK BREATHING FOR TEN SECONDS, *if no breathing*
BREATHE – *2 breaths*
ASSESS CIRCULATION *for 10 seconds*
START CHEST COMPRESSIONS *at 15 to every 2 breaths*
for adults

– THE WORLD'S YOUNGEST DOCTOR –

Dr Balamurali Ambati qualified as a doctor from the Mount S
School of Medicine in New York on 19 May 1995, at the
17 years 9 months and 21 days.

– THE MINI-MENTAL STATE EXAMINATION –

The Mini-Mental State Examination (MMSE) is a brief, quantitative measure of cognitive status in adults. Some sample items are as follows:

What day of the week is it?

What is the date today?

I am going to give you a piece of of paper – I want you to hold it in your right hand, fold it in half and place it on your lap

Show patient a pencil and ask what it is

Repeat after me: 'No ifs, ands, or buts'

Please read what is written and do what it says – 'CLOSE YOUR EYES'

Please copy this drawing

I am going to name three objects and I want you to say them back to me – I will ask you to remember them shortly.

Take 7 away from 100 and keep subtracting 7 until I ask you to stop

What were the three objects I mentioned a while ago?

Reproduced by special permission of the publisher, Psychological Assessment Resources Inc

– AN EXAMPLE OF A SNELLEN CHART TO ASSESS VISUAL ACUITY –

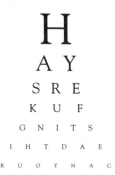

– CLINICAL AUDIT –

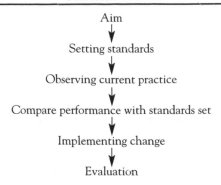

Aim
↓
Setting standards
↓
Observing current practice
↓
Compare performance with standards set
↓
Implementing change
↓
Evaluation

– THE MADNESS OF KING GEORGE –

King George III suffered from a rare condition called acute intermittent porphyria. It is an inherited metabolic disorder that affects the manufacture of haemoglobin. Recent groundbreaking research has shown that much of the medicine used to treat the King may have actually made his attacks much worse. Many medicines at the time contained arsenic, which has been shown to induce attacks of porphyria. Symptoms of an acute attack may include vomiting, fits, odd behaviour and the reddening of urine.

– CREATININE CLEARANCE –

Creatinine clearance (mL/min) =

$$\frac{(140 - \text{age in years}) \times (\text{weight in kg})}{72 \times \text{serum creatinine in mg/dL}}$$

Excreted by the kidney, creatinine is a breakdown product of creatine which is found in muscle. If kidney function is abnormal levels of creatinine will rise in the blood as the kidney is unab' to excrete it efficiently. Creatinine clearance is a measure of kid function and involves collecting urine for 24 hours and tal blood sample at the end of the 24 hours. It is an estimat volume of filtrate made by the kidney each minute.

– METHODS OF ADMINISTERING ANALGESIA –

Oral	Intravenous
Sublingual	Regional
Inhaled	Electrical
Intramuscular	

– THE NATO PHONETIC ALPHABET USED IN PRE-HOSPITAL COMMUNICATION BY AMBULANCE CREWS –

Alpha	Juliet	Sierra
Bravo	Kilo	Tango
Charlie	Lima	Uniform
Delta	Mike	Victor
Echo	November	Whisky
Foxtrot	Oscar	X-ray
Golf	Papa	Yankee
Hotel	Quebec	Zulu
India	Romeo	

– SOME RULES FOR AVOIDING JET LAG –

If you are flying westbound, avoid sleeping on the flight, as the day effectively lengthens

If you are flying eastbound (e.g. New York to London), sleep as much as possible on the flight

Daytime flights are the best for avoiding jet lag

Melatonin can help counter the effects of jet lag

– MEDICAL TERMS FOR TEMPERATURE RANGES –

Normal	36.6–37.2°C
Subnormal	<36.6°C
Febrile	>37.2°C
Hyperpyrexial	>41.6°C
Hypothermic	<35°C

– LORENZO'S OIL –

Lorenzo's Oil is a moving film portraying the true story of Augusto and Michaela Odone and their son, Lorenzo, who has a condition called adenoleukodystrophy (ADL). The condition is inherited and affects myelin – the lining of the spinal cord and nerves – leaving the affected patient severely disabled. The story of the oil is one of tireless effort on the part of the Odones, who proposed that erucic and oleic acid could reduce the levels of very long-chain fatty acids in the body – which are high in ADL. Augusto Odone is an economist and Michaela was an editor, and, unsurprisingly, there was dissent amongst physicians who felt threatened by these two non-medics proposing their theory. The couple eventually found help from a company in the UK who made the oil, and great debate continues about whether the oil actually helps patients with ADL. Many believe that it does, although scientific studies vary in opinion.

– SOME CONDITIONS AFFECTING BOTH HUMANS AND ANIMALS –

Allergies	Infertility
Asthma	Influenza
Botulism	Malaria
Cancer	Measles
Cardiovascular disease	Muscular dystrophy
Cataracts	Osteoarthritis
Cholera	Polio
Diabetes	Rabies
Diphtheria	Rheumatoid arthritis
Epilepsy	Rubella
Herpes virus	Tetanus
Hepatitis	Thyroiditis
Hypertension	Toxoplasmosis

– HEAD LICE –

Contrary to popular belief, head lice do not jump.

– SOME APPROXIMATE CONVERSIONS –

1 fluid ounce	28 mL
1 gallon	4.5 L
1 grain	65 mg
1 inch	25.4 mm
1 foot	0.3 m
1 ounce	28 g
1 pound	0.45 kg
1 calorie	4.2 J
1 kilocalorie	4.2 kJ

– HYPERSENSITIVITY REACTIONS –

Type I	Atopy and anaphylaxis
Type II	Cytotoxic hypersensitivity
Type III	Immune complex hypersensitivity
Type IV	Delayed-type hypersensitivity

– DI CLEMENTE AND PROCHASKA'S CYCLE OF CHANGE (FOR BEHAVIOURS) –

Pre-contemplation
↓
Contemplation
↓
Preparation
↓
Action
↓
Maintenance
↓
Relapse

– THE THIRD LARGEST EMPLOYER ON EARTH –

The UK National Health Service (NHS) is the third largest employer in the world after the Chinese Army and Indian Rail. It currently employs over 1.25 million people.

– APOTEMNOPHILIA –

Apotemnophilia is a kind of body dysmorphic syndrome in which people are convinced that they need to remove a limb in order to be normal. This belief usually starts in childhood and affected persons will go to extraordinary lengths to feel 'normal', such as shooting their own leg. A surgeon in Scotland removed limbs from two men for such a condition in the late 1990s.

– AMERICAN SOCIETY OF ANESTHETISTS (ASA) CLASSIFICATION OF A PATIENT'S CONDITION –

1 Normally healthy
2 Mild systemic disease
3 Severe systemic disease limiting activity; not incapacitating
4 Incapacitating systemic disease posing a threat to life
5 Moribund – not expected to survive 24 hours even with operation

– SOME WAYS OF DESCRIBING PERSONALITY DISORDERS –

Anankastic	Emotionally unstable
Antisocial	Histrionic
Avoidant	Narcissistic
Borderline	Obsessive-compulsive
Dependent	Paranoid
Dissocial	Schizoid

– SOME CAUSES OF ITCHING –

Eczema	Renal failure
Scabies	Anaemia
Lichen planus	Pregnancy
Dermatitis	Thyroid disorders
Drug reactions	Old age
Liver disease	

– ECONOMY CLASS SYNDROME –

Economy Class Syndrome is a modern term used to describe the theory that cramped seating on board long-haul international flights could lead to deep vein thrombosis (DVT) – a blood clot in a leg vein. It is generally recommended that passengers take aspirin before such flights to reduce the chance of this happening, although there is no medical evidence that it actually helps. Walking around should be encouraged during a flight to aid circulation in the legs. Other risk factors for DVT include the oral contraceptive pill and smoking. Economy Class Syndrome can apply to other forms of travel as well.

– TYPES OF CONTRACEPTION –

Intrauterine contraceptive device	Implant
Condom	Rhythm method
Cap	Pills
Diaphragm	Sterilization
Injection	

– SOME FAMOUS SUICIDES –

Kurt Cobain	Primo Levi
Ian Curtis	Harold Shipman
Adolf Hitler	Virginia Woolf
Judas Iscariot	Vincent Van Gogh

– THE LENGTH OF TIME THAT DRUGS LAST IN THE URINE –

Cocaine	24–48 hours
LSD	24–48 hours
Amphetamines	24–48 hours
Methadone	4 days
Benzodiazepines	Over a week
Heroin	48 hours
Cannabis	Up to 6 weeks

– SOME TRAVEL VACCINES –

Yellow fever	Meningococci
Typhoid	Japanese encephalitis
Tetanus	Tick encephalitis
Polio	Hepatitis A
Rabies	Hepatitis B

– GUYS' AND GIRLS' FIRST NAMES FOR SOME STREET DRUGS –

Drug	Name
Amphetamines	Billy
Cocaine	Charlie
Heroin	Harry
Marijuana	Mary

– FLATUS –

Flatus is the term given to gas in the intestine – or what is released when we pass wind. Every bit of flatus that leaves the body – i.e. through the passage of wind from the anus – always contains some liquid.

– SOME CONDITIONS THAT SOMETIMES GO TOGETHER –

Asthma and eczema
Uveitis and ankylosing spondylitis
Diabetes and hypothyroidism
Back pain and depression

– THE SEVEN AGES OF WOMAN –

1. Birth
2. Childhood
3. Menarche
4. Reproductive
5. Climacteric
6. Menopause
7. Post-menopause

– WHY DO WE MOVE EVERY FEW MINUTES IN OUR SLEEP? –

The reason we move around in our sleep is because our brain knows that if we stayed still, it would take less than one hour for the circulation to be cut off to the parts of the body in contact with the mattress. This would eventually lead to the skin becoming damaged (necrotic) and a pressure sore would appear from a lack of blood supply to that area.

– JAPANESE DRINKING HABITS –

In Japan up to 50% of people have a reaction to alcohol that can include facial flushing, a runny nose and low blood pressure. This is because of a deficiency of the enzyme aldehyde dehydrogenase, which is responsible for breaking down alcohol. The condition applies to other groups of people, including Chinese peoples and Native Americans. The interesting irony is that Japan is one of the world's biggest importers of Scotch whisky!

– SOME NURSES FROM THE BIG AND SMALL SCREEN –

Nurse Lt Evelyn Johnson (Kate Beckinsale) – *Pearl Harbor*

Hana (Juliette Binoche) – *The English Patient*

Tina Seabrook (Claire Goose) – *Casualty*

Carol Hathaway (Julianna Margulies) – *ER*

Chrissie Williams (Tina Hobley) – *Holby City*

Matron (Hattie Jacques) – *Carry on Nurse*

Nurse Gladys Emmanuel (Lynda Baron) – *Open All Hours*

Anji (Sunetra Sarker) – *No Angels*

Nurse Mills (Joanne Whalley) – *The Singing Detective*

Nurse Susan Ball (Barbara Windsor) – *Carry on Matron*

Nurse Betty (Renée Zellweger) – *Nurse Betty*

– MUNCHAUSEN'S SYNDROME –

This is a condition in which the person with the illness invents their symptoms, occasionally harms himself, demands powerful medicines and unnecessary operations, and usually self-discharges prematurely. These patients have complex personality disorders, which are usually impossible to treat. Often the patient will have been to numerous hospitals and will have argued with many a doctor and nurse. If a person gives false accounts or fakes symptoms of their child's illness rather than their own, the condition is called Munchausen's syndrome by proxy.

– THE FRENCH PARADOX –

As a nation France drinks twice as much alcohol as the UK per person and eats more dairy fat. Amazingly, they only have a third of the rate of heart disease compared with their neighbours across the channel. This paradox is likely to be because alcohol in moderation is protective against heart disease.

– BEAU'S LINES –

Most people have longitudinal ridges in their nails, (in line with the length of their fingers), but single ridges that run across all the nails of both hands at the same level are called Beau's Lines. This phenomenon usually occurs after a major illness as the nails stop growing temporarily.

– MOBILE PHONES AND HEALTH –

The effect on health of mobile phones has been debated for some years now and the jury is still out. One study has shown that heavy users are more likely to develop acoustic neuromas (benign brain tumours) and another reported a higher incidence of symptoms such as headache and fatigue. Children are now being encouraged to use text messages in preference to calling, and to use a phone with a low specific absorption rate (SAR). More studies are needed to ascertain the long-term effects of mobile phone use.

– TRICHOBEZOAR – 'RAPUNZEL SYNDROME' –

Trichobezoar is the name given to a ball of hair in the bowel. Hair is swallowed and can lodge itself in the digestive system, causing bowel obstruction. This requires surgery. Emotional problems can sometimes cause people to eat their hair, leading to this peculiar condition.

– HYPOCHONDRIACS –

Hypochondriacs are people who have a preoccupation with illness and serious disease based on their interpretation of symptoms. The word originates from 'hypochondrium', which is the term given to the upper left and right quadrants of the abdomen. These patients tend to persist with their health beliefs despite medical reassurance. Famous hypochondriacs include Woody Allen, Michael Jackson and Dr Samuel Johnson.

– RUSSELL'S SIGN –

This is a subtle clinical sign seen on the knuckles of bulimic patients, who make themselves sick after eating. It is a graze or scab, usually over the middle knuckle on one hand, made by the patient's teeth while sticking fingers down his or her throat.

– THALIDOMIDE –

Thalidomide was a drug developed in the 1960s in West Germany for use as a sleeping pill. At the time, the drug was given to many people, including pregnant women for morning sickness – arguably before its side-effects were fully known. Around 10,000 children were born with affected limbs as a result. The drug is used worldwide nowadays for treating cancer (particularly myeloma), for HIV ~atment and for certain cases of leprosy. It is a drug that must be ~ judiciously on the right patients for the appropriate condi- ~or example, in Brazil, over the past few years, there have ~es of thalidomide being used in pregnancy to treat leprosy, ~ knowledge that the drug causes limb defects.

– LEPROSY –

Leprosy is also known as Hansen's disease, after Gerhard Hansen, who discovered the bacterium *Mycoplasma leprae* in 1873, although the disease is thought to have been around for thousands of years. It is a disfiguring condition that primarily involves the skin, eyes and upper respiratory tract and has affected people in every continent the world over. Historically, leprosy has been associated with huge stigma and social exclusion, including in ancient times, when it was considered to be a divine curse. The first treatment for leprosy was a drug called dapsone in the 1940s, but bacterial resistance to this, and the growing use of antibiotic therapy, now means that leprosy is treated by multidrug therapy – a combination of powerful antibiotics. The countries with the most sufferers are India, Brazil and Nepal.

– THE MEDICAL ROOTS OF THE JACUZZI –

The Jacuzzis were a large Italian American family who made water pumps for industrial use in the early part of the 20th century. One of the Jacuzzi brothers had a son (b. 1941) who developed arthritis as a toddler, and the boy used to attend regular hydrotherapy sessions. Not wanting him to suffer while at home, the Jacuzzis adapted a pump that could be fitted to a bath. They initially received commercial orders from schools and hospitals. The invention went on to gain popularity with the rich and famous and soon became the domestic luxury item that we recognize today. The first self-contained Jacuzzi whirlpool bath was made in 1968.

– DUKES CLASSIFICATION –

The Dukes classification is used to classify cancer of the colon. It is related to prognosis:

Dukes A: The cancer is confined to the lining of the colon
Dukes B: The cancer has penetrated the colon wall
Dukes C: The cancer has spread to the lymph nodes
Dukes D: The cancer has spread to other organs

– BETTY FORD –

Betty Ford was the wife of former American President Gerald Ford and was committed to the treatment of addictions. She set up the Betty Ford Center in 1982 after dealing with her own chemical dependency and battling with breast cancer. The Center still runs today.

– MAD COW DISEASE –

'Mad cow disease' is the common name for bovine spongiform encephalopathy (BSE) and is a disease that affects cattle. BSE is a prion disease – one that results in an abnormal build-up of proteins in the brain. It takes up to six years for infected cattle to show signs of the disease, which can include aggressive behaviour and disorientation. Although the infection comes from animal brains, meat does not intentionally form part of normal cattle diet. The infected tissue is thought to have been contained in 'meat and bone meal', which is an artificial cattle feed. It is no longer made. The human equivalent of BSE is called Creutzfeldt–Jakob disease (CJD), which causes dementia – usually after the age of 40. Scientists discovered a new form of CJD in 1996 affecting people younger than this and named it 'variant' CJD (vCJD).

– A 66-YEAR-OLD GIVES BIRTH –

On 17 January 2005, 66-year-old Adriana Iliescu became the oldest woman recorded to give birth. She gave birth to a baby girl Eliza-Maria, who weighed 1.45 kilograms. The child's twin sister was stillborn. Professor Iliescu writes children's books for a living and used anonymous donor sperm for in vitro fertilization.

– THE LONE BONE –

hyoid bone is the only bone in the body not to be attached others. It is at the front of the neck above the 'Adam's yroid cartilage). Fracture of the hyoid is rare and is usu- g after death by strangulation.

– ANAESTHETIC AWARENESS –

Anaesthetic awareness is a rare phenomenon in which a patient under anaesthetic is able to recall details from the operation. It was first studied in the 1960s. There are two types of awareness – implicit and explicit – the latter being more traumatic when on occasion every word and action from the operating theatre can be recalled. The implicit type usually presents afterwards as odd dreams, nightmares, sleep disturbances, anxiety or flashbacks. Some patients develop a preoccupation with death. A small minority of patients may develop post-traumatic stress disorder. The estimate of the frequency of anaesthetic awareness varies, but is 1% or less. Interestingly, a recent study showed that patients who dream under anaesthetic are likely to be less satisfied with their care.*

(*Leslie K et al, Dreaming during anaesthesia in patients at high risk of awareness. *Anaesthesia*, March 2005, vol 60, 239)

– BOOB JOBS –

For many years after the Second World War, Japanese prostitutes had tried augmenting their breasts with paraffin and non-medical silicone. Modern breast augmentation was invented in 1962 by plastic surgeons Thomas Cronin and Frank Gerow at the University of Texas, USA. It was intended originally for patients who had had mastectomies (breast removal for cancer), but quickly became popular with the rest of the population. Nowadays, saline implants are used in preference to silicone implants, which have caused problems with local scarring and rupture.

– HOT WATER BOTTLES –

Erythema ab igne is the name given to the reddening skin seen on the legs or the abdomen of people who are regularly in contact with a hot water bottle. The skin has a characteristic appearance and people, usually elderly, often consult their doctor about rash. The same can happen from sitting in front of a fire.

– LEG LENGTHENING –

In China today, people who would like to be taller spend large amounts of money on having their legs lengthened by orthopaedic surgery. Recovery is slow and painful and can take the best part of a year.

– SAD –

Seasonal affective disorder or SAD is a condition in which sufferers feel low because of the time of year and low light levels. The 'winter blues' affect about 2% of the UK population and up to 10% of Americans. Treatment is with antidepressants or light boxes that can re-create natural light. SAD is not the only medical phenomenon associated with a lack of light. 'Sundowning' is a colloquial term given to the temporary evening-time agitation that affects hospital and community patients (particularly the elderly) as daylight fades.

– MEDICINAL AND HARMFUL EFFECTS OF CANNABIS, AS STUDIED –

Can relieve nausea

Can lower blood pressure

Can reduce pressure in glaucoma

Can relieve some types of pain

Can relieve bronchospasm

Can cause cancer

Can cause bronchitis

Can cause psychosis

– DEATH BY COCONUT –

\>roximately 75 tourists and travellers a year are killed every
\>y coconuts falling from trees.

– THE ANALGESIA LADDER FOR TREATING PAIN –

Paracetamol, aspirin, ibuprofen

↓

Dextropropoxyphene, dihydrocodeine, codeine, tramadol

↓

Diamorphine, morphine, fentanyl, methadone

– SOME APHRODISIAC FOODS –

Bananas	Carrots
Mussels	Truffles
Asparagus	Chocolate
Onions	Oysters

– SOME HEALTH BENEFITS OF GARLIC (*ALLIUM SATIVUM*) –

Lowers blood pressure	Anti-yeast properties
Lowers cholesterol	Antibacterial properties
Anticancer properties	

– MRSA –

Amazingly, methicillin-resistant *Staphylococcus aureus* (MRSA) is most commonly carried totally harmlessly by people. It can, of course, cause serious illness in susceptible people. Rigorous hand washing and wearing gloves in hospitals can help stop it from spreading.

– THE LONGEST COMA –

The longest recorded coma lasted for over 37 years. Americ͟ Elaine Esposito had an operation to remove her appendix in 1͟ at the age of six, after which she failed to regain consciou͟ She died in November 1978, aged 43.

– FAMOUS PEOPLE CURRENTLY OR PREVIOUSLY MARRIED TO DOCTORS –

Clive Anderson	Vanessa Feltz
JK Rowling	Sir Steve Redgrave
Sachin Tendulkar	Natascha McElhone
Robin Cook	Baroness Jay

– MISS PLASTIC SURGERY –

In China there is an annual beauty contest exclusively for women who have had plastic surgery. Each entrant must produce a letter from a doctor as proof that they have undergone plastic surgery before being allowed to compete.

– HUNGRY HIPPOS –

Despite their cute image and media iconoclasm in the form of cuddly toys, cartoon characters and sweets, hippopotamuses are responsible for the most human deaths by any mammal each year.

– SURVIVING A FREE FALL OF OVER 30,000 FEET WITHOUT A PARACHUTE –

This is exactly what record-breaking air stewardess Vesna Vulovic did in 1972 when her JAT (Jugoslavenski Aerotransport) flight exploded in mid-air, apparently due to a terrorist bomb. She landed in deep snow, broke both of her legs, but miraculously survived.

– OTTAWA ANKLE RULE –

Ankle injuries are very common in emergency departments. The Ottawa rules were developed in 1992 to avoid unnecessary X-rays. An X-ray of the ankle is needed only if there is bony tenderness at the tip or posterior edge of either malleolus or the patient is unable to bear weight immediately after injury and in the Emergency Department.

– THE INDEX-RING DIFFERENTIAL –

The difference in length between the ring and index finger on your hand is supposed to be of great significance according to some psychologists. The greater the difference in length, the more likely that person is to be an entrepreneur, take risks and be highly successful. That person is also more likely to have a one-night stand, likely to want a life less ordinary than others and more likely to have sociopathic tendencies.

– THE FIRST TEST-TUBE BABY –

The first test-tube baby was Louise Brown, who was delivered by Caesarean section in Oldham, Lancashire on 25 July 1978. She weighed 2.6 kg at birth.

Interestingly, some of the first fertility drugs, such as Pergonal®, were made from the urine of post-menopausal nuns, a substance that is naturally rich in FSH (follicle-stimulating hormone) and LH (luteinising hormone). Both hormones effectively encourage ovulation.

– GENUINE REASONS WHY PEOPLE HAVE CALLED AN EMERGENCY AMBULANCE (UK) –

Toothache	Stubbed toe
For an 'annual check-up'	Run out of paracetamol
Split condom	Wanting to be put in to bed
Hiccups	A broken nail

– THE ORIGINAL SIAMESE TWINS –

The term 'Siamese' refers to twins connected by living tissue. The original 'Siamese twins' were Chang and Eng, born in 1811 in Melange in Siam. At the time, the king of Siam (Rama II) initially decided that the babies should be put to death. He eventually changed his mind. As teenagers, the twin boys were brought to England briefly before settling in the USA, where they both had families and lived until their death in 1874.

– FOLIE À DEUX –

This is a rare and fascinating psychiatric condition in which two people suffer from almost exactly the same delusion or abnormal belief. It is more common when the two persons live in isolation and in close proximity to each other. The condition can affect more than two people, even whole families.

– SOME TRIGGERS FOR MIGRAINE –

Chocolate	Hunger
Fatigue	Noise
Wine	Bright lights
Caffeine	Stress
Citrus fruits	

– HEART MURMURS AND THEIR POSSIBLE CAUSES –

Murmur	Possible causes
Ejection systolic	Flow murmur, aortic stenosis, pulmonary stenosis, hypertrophic obstructive cardiomyopathy
Pansystolic	Mitral regurgitation, tricuspid regurgitation, ventral septal defect, atrial septal defect
Early diastolic	Aortic regurgitation, pulmonary regurgitation, tricuspid stenosis
Mid-diastolic	Mitral stenosis, aortic regurgitation

– NORMAL PARAMETERS OF SEMEN ANALYSIS –

pH	7.2–8.0
Volume	2.0 mL
Sperm count	>20 x 10^6 spermatozoa/mL
Motility	> 50% with forward progression or 25% with rapid progression
Normal forms	< 50%

– TYPES OF THYROID CANCER –

Papillary	Medullary
Follicular	Lymphoma
Anaplastic	

– HYSTERIA –

Hysteria was originally believed to be a psychological state affecting women and resulting from a disturbance in the uterus. The word root *hyster-* comes from the Greek word for womb (hence 'hysterectomy' means the 'removal of the womb'). The phrase was first coined in the 17th century.

– MEDICINES –

The definition of a medicine or medicinal substance in the UK by the 1968 Medicines Act is one that alters physiological processes and is used for the treatment of illness, for anaesthesia, for contraception, for maintaining health or as a test for diagnosing illness.

– THE PHASES OF CLINICAL TRIALS –

Phase I	Clinical pharmacology in volunteers
Phase II	Small-scale studies (small numbers of patients)
Phase III	Large-scale trials (thousands of patients)
Phase IV	Surveillance to evaluate safety and efficacy
Phase V	Further trials

– ETHICAL CONSIDERATIONS IN MEDICINE –

Autonomy
Beneficence
Consent and Confidentiality
Do no harm
Equity

– ROLES WITHIN A TEAM (BELBIN®) –

Coordinator
Shaper
Plant
Resource investigator
Implementer
Monitor evaluator
Teamworker
Completer finisher
Specialist

– MONSIEUR MANGETOUT –

Michel Lotito is also known as Monsieur Mangetout. Since childhood he has eaten an odd diet of numerous materials that are not digestible. These include metal and glass and even a whole light aircraft (a Cessna 150), which took him almost two years to finish. Doctors have found that he has an unusually thick bowel wall but cannot explain his digestive tolerance to these materials, which would normally be harmful.

– HANDICAP –

The commonly held belief is that the word 'handicap' is derived from 'hand in cap', suggesting that historically handicapped people had to beg for a living. In fact the word probably comes from betting and racing circles in the early part of the 20th century, when horses had to be handicapped or disabled to a degree with weights in order to even up the odds during a race.

– SOME FAMOUS INSOMNIACS –

Napoleon Bonaparte
Sir Winston Churchill
Charles Dickens
Thomas Edison
Marcel Proust

Vincent Van Gogh
Benjamin Franklin
Cary Grant
Marilyn Monroe

– MORAL THEORIES –

Theory of virtue	Theory of utility
Theory of duties	Theory of rights

– PAVLOV'S DOGS –

Ivan Pavlov (1849–1936) was a Russian physiologist famous for his landmark study on classical conditioning, which is a learnt behaviour. His dogs expected food at a certain time when he entered their room, and would start to salivate in expectation. He coupled the sound of a bell with feeding them (providing a neutral stimulus – i.e. something that would not usually make the dogs salivate). Eventually, after this was repeated numerous times, the sound of the bell alone was enough to make the dogs salivate. This showed that the animal brain could be trained (or conditioned) to respond to a stimulus based on the outcomes of previous experience.

– SOME DIFFERENT KINDS OF GENETIC DISEASES –

Autosomal dominant
Marfan's syndrome
Otosclerosis

Autosomal recessive
Cystic fibrosis
Sickle cell anaemia
Thalassaemia

X-linked dominant
Coffin-Lowry syndrome
Incontinentia pigmenti

X-linked recessive
Duchenne muscular dystrophy
Fragile-X syndrome
Haemophilia
Red–green colour deficiency

– A POPULAR 'SIEVE'/AIDE-MEMOIRE USED BY MEDICAL STUDENTS –

Dressed In A Surgeon's Gown A Physician Might Make Some Progress

(Definition/ Incidence/ Age/ Sex/ Geography/ Aetiology/ Pathology/Micro/Macro Symptoms and signs/ Prognosis)

– SOME POSSIBLE HANGOVER REMEDIES –

Berocca®
Caffeine
Water
Salt solution
Fruit juices
Eggs
Cheese
Cabbage
Alcohol (hair of the dog)
A hot shower
A cold shower
A hot shower followed by a cold shower
Isotonic drinks
Sticking your head in a fridge
N-acetylcysteine (NAC)
Oxygen
Acupressure
'Resolve'
Massage

– DRUGS THAT MAY CAUSE GYNAECOMASTIA* –

Digoxin
Isoniazid
Spironolactone
Cimetidine
Oestrogen

*nlargement of the male breast

– TOP TEN GLOBAL CAUSES OF MORTALITY (IN ORDER) –

Ischaemic heart disease and stroke

Lower respiratory tract infections

HIV/AIDS

Chronic obstructive pulmonary disease

Diarrhoeal diseases

Tuberculosis

Childhood illnesses

Cancer of lung, trachea and bronchus

Road traffic accidents

Malaria

– HAIR AND NAILS –

On average, the hair on our heads grows at 11 mm per month and nails grow at 3 mm per month.

– EYE JEWELLERY –

Dutch surgeons have created a piece of jewellery (JewelEye®) that can be inserted underneath the conjunctiva of the eye. There are as yet no side effects and the half moon or heart-shaped pieces are clearly visible on the eye.

– SPERM WASHING –

Sperm washing is a technique that involves removing sperm from seminal fluid and placing it in a nutrient to enhance its motility. This is often done in intrauterine insemination, a technique used to treat infertility, as well as in men with HIV. This allows the chance for an HIV-positive man to have a baby without risk to it or the mother, as the virus is thought only to be carried in the seminal fluid and not the sperm itself.

– NAZI MEDICAL EXPERIMENTS –

In complete contrast to the premise of the medical profession, which is to help and to 'do no harm', Nazi doctors during the Third Reich carried out some horrific and unethical medical experiments on their victims. These included including freezing to explore hypothermia, infecting victims to test immunizations, burning and boiling victims, mass sterilization, and torture. Genetic experiments were carried out as well.

– APOTHECARIES' WEIGHTS –

This is a traditional system of weight used in the UK for measuring and dispensing pharmaceuticals. 20 grains equal 1 scruple; 3 scruples equal 1 dram; 8 drams equal 1 apothecary's ounce (oz apoth.), and 12 such ounces equal one apothecary's pound (lb apoth.).

– SOME DRUG GROUPS ASSOCIATED WITH ERECTILE DYSFUNCTION –

Antipsychotics
Antihypertensives
Anticholinergics
Antiandrogens

Antidepressants
Dopamine anatagonists
H2 antagonists

– CONDITIONS IN WHICH ANTINUCLEAR ANTIBODIES (ANA) ARE FOUND –

Systemic lupus erythematosus
Scleroderma
Sjögren's syndrome
Rheumatoid arthritis
Chronic active hepatitis

Chronic infections
Old age
Polymyositis
Dermatomyositis

Antinuclear antibodies are abnormal antibodies that work against the body's tissues, i.e. 'autoantibodies'. We all have some autoantibodies, but approximately 5% of people have a large amount, and, as such, have more of a propensity for developing an autoimmune condition, some of which are listed above.

– SOME FOODS AND DRINKS CONTAINING OXALATE (WHICH CAN BE A CAUSE OF KIDNEY STONES) –

Chocolate	Nuts	Strawberries
Coffee	Rhubarb	Tea
Cola	Spinach	

– RING A RING O' ROSES –

The 'roses' in this popular nursery rhyme referring to the rosy rash, which was one of the symptoms of the Great Plague of 1665. The 'pocketful of posies' was a bunch of herbs used to fight off the illness. 'A-tishoo, a-tishoo' refers to sneezing in the final stage of the illnees, and 'We all fall down' refers to death.

– GOING DOOLALLY –

It may not sound it, but the word 'Doolally' has its origins in India during the time of British rule. It comes from the name Deolali, a small town near Mumbai, where British soldiers were sent after their tours of duty, awaiting transfer home. Often these men would be isolated, sometimes for many months and would be described as having 'Doolally tap' – meaning odd behaviour or temporary insanity brought about by being in Deolali. This later evolved into 'going Doolally'.

– JOHN SNOW AND SANITATION IN SOHO, LONDON –

Dr John Snow was the first person to carry out a substantial epidemiological study – that is the study of the distribution, spread and occurrence of disease. He managed to link deaths from an outbreak of cholera in London in 1854 to a water pump in Broad Street, Soho. People had been drinking cold water from it during the heat of the summer rather than boiling it for tea. Removal of the pump saw a dramatic decrease in the death rate. This study had huge impact on the future sanitation and sewerage of London.

– SOME DRUGS WITH A NARROW THERAPEUTIC INDEX –

Lithium
Digoxin
Phenytoin
Carbamazepine
Cyclosporin

The therapeutic index of a drug is the ratio between the toxic dose and the therapeutic dose of a drug. It is used as a measure of the relative safety of the drug for a particular treatment. In simple terms, if the dose is too low, they will not have a therapeutic effect at all, and if the dose is too high, toxic side-effects may be experienced. With the drugs listed above, the difference in dose between delivering too little or too much of the drug is particularly narrow.

– CERVICAL INTRAEPITHELIAL NEOPLASIA (CIN) –

This is a histological diagnosis, usually following an abnormal smear test:

CIN I: Mild dysplasia – nuclear atypia confined to the basal third of the epithelium

CIN II: Moderate dysplasia – nuclear atypia confined to the basal two-thirds of the epithelium

CIN III: Severe dysplasia – nuclear atypia through the full thickness of the epithelium

CIN I to CIN III is a grading system related to the depth of the lining of the cervix to which abnormal cells appear. Many women with CIN I will find that their smears return to normal on their own. With CIN II and III there is some risk of progression to cervical cancer, but only over many years – usually in severe cases of CIN III that are left untreated. Treatments include laser therapy, cold coagulation, cryotherapy, a large loop excision, diathermy and cone biopsy, all of which either destroy or remove the abnormal cells.

– OLD ORIENTALIST GEOGRAPHICAL COLLOQUIALISMS FOR TRAVELLER'S DIARRHOEA –

Aztec Two-Step	Turkey's Trots
Delhi Belly	Gippy Tummy (Egypt)
Karachi Cork	Hong Kong Dog
Rangoon Runs	Kathmandu Quickstep
Montezuma's Revenge	

– ORGANS SUITABLE FOR DONATION AFTER DEATH –

Skin	Cornea
Bone	Heart valves

– GLYCAEMIC INDEX OF FOODS (GI) –

Only foods that contain carbohydrates have a glycaemic index (GI). GI is a measure of how fast each food has an effect on raising blood glucose. Pure glucose has the most dramatic effect and hence has a GI of 100. Below is a list of foods and their corresponding glycaemic indices. Foods with a GI below 55 can aid weight loss.

Peanuts	14	Bananas	55
Grapefruit	25	Pitta bread	57
Red lentils	26	Basmati rice	58
Whole milk	27	Digestive biscuit	59
Low-fat fruit yoghurt	33	Cheese and tomato pizza	60
Apples and pears	38	Ice cream	61
Tomato soup, canned	38	New potatoes	62
Apple juice	40	Cola	63
Noodles and white pasta	40	Croissants	67
Chick peas (canned)	42	Wholemeal bread	69
Oranges	44	Mashed potato	70
Green grapes	46	White bread	70
Peas	48	French fries	75
Baked beans	48	Jelly beans	80
Carrots, boiled	49	Cornflakes	84
Milk chocolate	49	Jacket potatoes	85
Crisps	54	Parsnips (boiled)	97

– SOME FACTS ABOUT THE COMMON COLD –

Colds last on average for one week but they can last just a few days or up to two weeks.

Children's noses are the main source of cold viruses.

There are over 100 different cold viruses. Rhinoviruses cause at least one-half of colds.

Cold viruses live only in the noses of humans and chimpanzees or other higher primates – not in other animals.

There is no cure for the common cold.

– DR KELLOGG AND CORNFLAKES –

Dr John Harvey Kellogg was a surgeon with a special interest in nutrition. He originally created cornflakes with the help of his brother William in Michigan in 1898. He intended cornflakes to be taken regularly as part of a diet to lessen sex drive and prevent the urge to masturbate, as well as being good for the bowel. Kellogg believed that health and illness was related to the health of the colon. He and his brother both lived until the age of 91 years.

– LACTOBACILLI –

This is a group of 'friendly bacteria'. This means that they actually help protect us from disease. They have a number of beneficial effects, including the production of nutrients (vitamins B and K), providing energy through the production of short-chain fatty acids and protecting us from harmful bacteria by 'competing' with them.

– TNM CLASSIFICATION FOR MALIGNANT TUMOURS –

The TNM classification for staging cancers is internationally recognized and helps clinicians to plan treatment. It also gives an indication on prognosis. T is for primary Tumour, N is for regional lymph Nodes and M is for distant Metastases.

– SOME PROVEN HERBAL REMEDIES FOR SPECIFIC CONDITIONS –

Saw palmetto	Benign prostatic hypertrophy
Horse chestnut seeds	Chronic venous insufficiency
Agnus castus extract	Premenstrual syndrome
Black cohosh	Premenopausal symptoms
Gingko biloba	Dementia
Ginger	Motion sickness
Tea tree oil	Fungal infections
Hypericum (St John's wort)	Depression

– THE STORY BEHIND WARFARIN –

How did we humans ever come to take something medicinal that is used to kill rats? In the early part of the 20th century, farmers with silos noticed that their cattle were dying without good reason. Veterinary surgeons discovered that the animals had died of internal bleeding, presumably having fed on the silage. The hay from the silo contained a chemical called coumarin, and this, under the action of heat, moisture and pressure led to the formation of an anticoagulant. In order to study doses for human therapy, the drug was tried out as a rat poison (rodenticide). The name warfarin was derived from Wisconsin Alumni Research Foundation. Patients take warfarin for various conditions, including atrial fibrillation and deep vein thrombosis. It is monitored by a blood test called INR (International Normalized Ratio), which essentially is a measure of the clotting ability of the blood medicated with warfarin compared with normal blood.

– EUTHANASIA –

Euthanasia is a concept whereby health care professionals are able to end a patient's life, most often at the patient's request. The Netherlands was the first country to legalize euthanasia, in 2002. This is by no means a 'licence to kill' – there is a code that must be followed, including consultation with at least one other doctor.

– TINNITUS –

Tinnitus is a condition in which noise is heard inside the ear or head without any external source. It can be caused by external, middle or inner ear problems, including wax, infection, exposure to noise or drugs, but in many cases there is no obvious cause. The actual sensation of sound is caused by discharging nerve fibres which have a 'faulty connection' with the hair cells in the cochlea (inner ear). Tinnitus can resolve itself, and treatments include relaxation and masking devices.

– AIRBAGS –

Airbags have been available since the late 1980s in the USA, but were actually invented in 1953. The reason for this delay was the technological difficulty in distinguishing between a serious crash and a minor collision. In recent years there has been worry over the safety of airbags in terms of causing injury, particularly if deployed without a seatbelt. Studies vary regarding the effectiveness of airbags.

– MMR –

There has been much controversy around the safety of the combined MMR (measles, mumps, rubella) vaccine after a question was raised about whether it may cause autism or inflammatory bowel disease in a study by Dr Andrew Wakefield published in 1998 in *The Lancet*. There have been other studies since, and the weight of evidence that the combined MMR vaccine is actually safe is now considerable, at the time of writing.

– DOCTORS AS NATIONAL LEADERS –

Most doctors need leadership skills – some more than others. Ibrahim Al-Jafaari became the Prime Minister of Iraq in 2005, having worked as a GP in North London. He was born in Karbala, Iraq and educated at the University of Mosul. Also in the Middle East, Bashar al-Assad, an ophthalmologist, became Syria's president in 2000.

– H. PYLORI –

Spiral in shape, *Helicobacter pylori* is a flagellate bacterium (i.e. it is a bacterium with hair-like processes) that lives in the stomach and duodenum. It is able to protect itself from strong stomach acid by covering itself in the mucus that lines the stomach and by using an enzyme called urease to create bicarbonate and ammonia, which combat the acid. Almost two-thirds of the world's population are infected with the bacterium, although many people have no symptoms. The commonest health concern associated with *H. pylori* is that it can lead to ulcers in the stomach and duodenum. In patients with ulcers or symptoms of ulcers, eradicating the bacterium with treatment can prevent recurrence. *Helicobacter* is also found in cats and dogs.

– HOW LOUD ARE COMMON THINGS IN DECIBELS (dBA)? –

Sound	(dBA)
Inaudible	0
Just audible	10
Whispering at 5 feet	20
Soft whisper	30
Average living room	40
Refrigerator	50
Normal conversation	60
Noisy bar	70
Hairdryer	80
Tractor	90
Home lawnmower	100
Baby crying	110
Pneumatic drill	120
Rocket launch pad	180

Permanent damage to the ears can occur after prolonged exposure to noise above just 85 decibels, and after just ten minutes at 110 decibels.

– CURRENT CAREER STRUCTURE FOR DOCTORS IN THE UK –

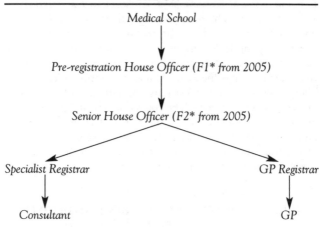

Medical School

↓

Pre-registration House Officer (F1* from 2005)

↓

Senior House Officer (F2* from 2005)

Specialist Registrar   *GP Registrar*

↓   ↓

Consultant   GP

* Foundation Year 1 and Foundation Year 2.

– MASLOW'S HIERARCHY OF NEEDS –

Physiological

Safety

Love

Esteem

Cognitive

Aesthetic

Self-actualization

(Maslow A, *Motivation and Personality*, 2nd edn (1970). New York, Harper & Row)

– THE BRAIN –

The brain weighs around 1.4 kg and contains over 100 billion cells. It receives about 20% of the blood from the heart.

– INDEX –